# National Health and Nutrition Examination Survey

# ANTHROPOMETRY AND PHYSICAL ACTIVITY MONITOR PROCEDURES MANUAL

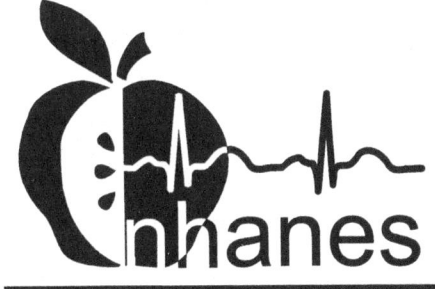

nhanes

January 2005

# TABLE OF CONTENTS

**TABLE OF CONTENTS (continued)**

# TABLE OF CONTENTS (continued)

List of Appendixes

List of Tables

List of Exhibits

# TABLE OF CONTENTS (continued)

## List of Exhibits (continued)

**TABLE OF CONTENTS (continued)**

List of Exhibits (continued)

# 1. INTRODUCTION TO ANTHROPOMETRY

## 1.1 Overview of Anthropometry

Nutrition is a major determinant of health, and the resolution of many nutritional issues of public health concern requires survey data. One of the major aims of NHANES is to provide information useful for studying the relationship among diet, nutritional status, and health. In addition to dietary intake methodologies, questionnaire material, hematological tests, and nutritional biochemistries, the assessment of nutritional status requires a series of stature, weight, and other anthropometric dimensions.

Anthropometry is the study of the measurement of the human body in terms of the dimensions of bone, muscle, and adipose (fat) tissue. Measures of subcutaneous adipose tissue are important because individuals with large values are reported to be at increased risks for hypertension, adult-onset diabetes mellitus, cardiovascular disease, gallstones, arthritis, various forms of cancer, and other diseases. Combined with the dietary and related questionnaire data, and the biochemical determinations, anthropometry is essential and critical information needed to assist in describing the data collected from persons in the NHANES sample.

## 1.2 Purpose of Anthropometrics

Actual stature, weight, and body measurements (including skinfolds and circumferences) will be collected in the MEC for purposes of assessing growth, body fat distribution, and for the provision of reference data. Anthropometric measurements such as skinfolds and circumferences, combined with Dual Energy X-Ray Absorptiometry (DXA), will allow analysis of the relationship between obesity and risk of disease. Therefore, many of the measurements included in NHANES will repeat ones made in previous NHANES and HHANES surveys so that trend analyses can be conducted. One measure has been added to provide further information on body frame size, while others have been dropped because new data have determined that other measures are more informative.

## 1.3 Role of Anthropometric Examiner and Recorder

The collection of anthropometric data require an examiner and recorder. Health technologists for NHANES will be trained to perform both roles. In addition, other MEC staff will be trained to serve as recorders. It is important when two health technologists are in the room that the examiner assigned to the room complete the examination once it is started.

The examiner will be responsible for positioning the SP, taking each measurement, and stating the measurement aloud to the recorder. The recorder will enter it into the automated system, and if there is no out-of-range message, state the name of the next measurement listed on the computer screen. With the exception of skinfolds, the examiner should keep the measuring instrument set on the SP until the recorder enters the number and the computer repeats it. If there is an out-of-range message, the recorder will repeat the entry and the examiner will check it. The recorder will change the number ONLY if the number the examiner read was incorrect.

It is the recorder's role to "assist" the examiner in obtaining correct measurements. This includes helping the examiner correctly position the SP and checking to make sure the SP is standing or sitting erect for specified measurements, and that the SP is holding onto appropriate bars for support during specified measures. During the examination, it will be the recorder's responsibility to make the midpoint marks on the SP. The recorder will also assist the examiner by checking the tension and horizontal position of the steel measuring tape for girth measurements.

# 2. EQUIPMENT

## 2.1  Description of Exam Room in MEC

The body measurement room is located in trailer #4 of the MEC. The room is equipped with some unique features designed to facilitate an accurate and efficient measurement procedure. These features include strategically placed mirrors and a custom-built box for SPs to sit on. In addition, the Toledo scale, stadiometer, and infantometer (infant measurement board) are supported by the Integrated Survey Information System (ISIS) for quick and accurate data capture.

## 2.2  Description of Equipment and Supplies

The equipment and supplies necessary for body measurements are as follows:

- Toledo electronic weight scale
- Seca electronic stadiometer
- Seca electronic infantometer
- Measurement box for upper leg length and calf circumference
- Insertion tape
- Steel measuring tape
- Holtain skinfold caliper
- Holtain small sliding breadth caliper
- Computer terminal

- Weights for scale calibration
- Calibration rods
- Step wedge standards
- Cosmetic pencils (wax base)
- Scissors - blunt edge
- Masking tape
- Baby oil
- Gauze 4x4
- Seca digital scales (2)

### 2.2.1  Inventory of Equipment and Supplies

At the beginning and end of each stand, the health technologist should take an inventory of the equipment and supplies needed for the body measurement examination component as discussed in Standardized Procedures. Any pieces of equipment that are missing should be reported to the MEC manager.

## 2.3    Start of Stand Procedures

Unpack the equipment and supplies and arrange accordingly in the room. Clean and calibrate the equipment as discussed in this chapter.

### 2.3.1    Equipment and Setup Procedures

You will need to unpack all the supplies and equipment before starting the first session of the new stand. The procedures are described in this section.

#### 2.3.1.1    Supplies

- Take the stick out of the drawer handles and store in the anthropometry storage box.

- Remove the supplies (e.g., alcohol, gauze pads, cosmetic pencils) and equipment (e.g., small sliding calipers, skinfold calipers, head circumference tape) from the drawers and put them in the baskets mounted on the walls.

- Hang a small plastic bag (found in the second drawer) on the hook under the desk for discarding soiled gauze, cotton, etc.

#### 2.3.1.2    Weights

- Remove the filler from around the weights and store in the anthropometry storage box.

- Remove the weight gate and store in the anthropometry storage box.

#### 2.3.1.3    Measurement Box

- Remove the strap from around the box and the foam pad from behind the box, and store in the anthropometry storage box.

**2.3.1.4    Digital Weight Scale**

■    Lift the cover off the scale and check that all four feet of the base are on the metal platform.

■    Adjust the scale if needed and return the cover to the scale.

**2.3.1.5    Stadiometer**

■    Remove the strap from the sitting box and move to the opposite wall. Store the strap in the anthropometry storage box. Push the headpiece of the stadiometer to the top of the measurement column, place the strap (stored in anthropometry storage box) around the headpiece, and attach the strap to the hooks in the wall.

**2.3.1.6    Infantometer**

■    Remove the strap from the infantometer and store it in the anthropometry storage box.

**2.3.2    Calibration Procedures**

Four pieces of equipment will be calibrated at the start of the stand by the technologist assigned to the anthropometry room. They include the scale, the infantometer, the stadiometer, and the skinfold calipers. The calibration procedures for each piece of equipment are described below.

**2.3.2.1    Digital Weight Scale**

■    Place all six of the 50-pound calibrated weights on the scale and capture the weight in the QC Checks dialog box, Start of Stand tab. Click the Done box corresponding to the scale when the calibration is complete.

■    The acceptable range for the scale is 299.75-300.25. If it weighs outside this range, notify the MEC manager to have the scale recalibrated by a service representative.

### 2.3.2.2    Infantometer

- Move the footboard with the digital display to the head of the infantometer as far as it will go. In MEC 1, the digital display should read 16 cm. In MECs 2 and 3, the digital display should read 0 cm.

- Capture the counter reading in the QC Checks Start of Stand dialog box. Click the Done box corresponding to the infantometer when the calibration is complete. If the infantometer is not measuring correctly, you will need to recalibrate it.

- To recalibrate, adjust the digital display reading to read 16 cm or 0 cm by pressing the + or - button on the infantometer footboard. Note in the comment box that the infantometer was recalibrated to 16 or 0.


### 2.3.2.3    Stadiometer

- Place the calibration rod on the floor of the stadiometer.

- Place the horizontal bar of the stadiometer firmly against the top of the calibration rod. The digital display should read 80 cm.

- Capture the counter reading in the QC Checks Start of Stand dialog box. Click the Done box corresponding to the stadiometer when the calibration is complete. If the stadiometer display does not read 80 cm, you will need to recalibrate it.

- To recalibrate, adjust the stadiometer headpiece digital display reading to read 80 cm by pressing the + or the - button. Note in the comment box that the stadiometer was recalibrated to 80 cm.


### 2.3.2.4    Skinfold Calipers

- Zero the calipers before starting the calibration procedures. Place the step wedge standard between the caliper arms at each of the four steps, and check that the reading falls within the acceptable range.

- Record the measurement taken at each step in the Quality Control Checks Result field. An identical calibration should be done on the spare set of skinfold calipers and the corresponding measurements also recorded in the QC Checks Result field. Click the Done box corresponding to the skinfold calipers when the calibration is complete.

- If the caliper readings fall outside the acceptable range at any level, use the other set of calipers and inform the MEC manager. They will be returned to the manufacturer for adjustment.

- If the calipers become too loose, use the spare set of calipers and inform the MEC manager.

- The acceptable ranges for the step wedge readings are as follows:

| | | | |
|---|---|---|---|
| first step | 9.8 – 10.5 | third step | 29.9 – 30.5 |
| second step | 19.8 – 20.5 | fourth step | 39.8 – 40.4 |

### 2.3.2.5 Seca Digital Scale

- Place the scale on the floor and activate it by lightly touching the surface with your foot.

- Verify that the scale is set to measure weight in pounds by checking the switch on the back of the scale.

- Wait for the display to read 0.0.

- Carefully place five of the 50-pound weights on the scale, for a total of 250 pounds.

- Read the result when the digital display has stabilized.

- The acceptable weight range for the full calibration is 248.8 – 251.0 pounds.

- If the scale weighs outside the acceptable range, inform the MEC manager. The home office will be contacted and replacement scales will be sent.

### 2.4 Mid-Stand Calibration Procedures

Calibrate the scale using the same procedures as those for Start of Stand Calibration.

- Place all six of the 50 pound calibrated weights on the scale and capture the weight in the QC Checks dialog box, Start of Stand tab. Click the Done box corresponding to the scale when the calibration is complete.

- If there is any reason to believe that the scale is not accurate, notify the data manager to recalibrate the scale.

### 2.5 Weekly Calibration Procedures

Three pieces of equipment will be calibrated weekly: the infantometer, stadiometer, and skinfold calipers. The calibration procedures are described below.

### 2.5.1    Infantometer

■    Follow the same procedures as for start of stand. Move the footboard with the digital display to the head of the infantometer as far as it will go. The digital display should read 16 cm in MEC 1; in MECs 2 and 3, the digital display should read 0 cm.

■    Capture the counter reading in the QC Checks Weekly dialog box. Click the Done box corresponding to the infantometer when the calibration is complete. If the infantometer is not measuring correctly, you will need to recalibrate it.

■    To recalibrate, adjust the digital display reading to read 16 cm or 0 cm by pressing the + or - button on the infantometer footboard. Note in the comment box that the infantometer was recalibrated to 16 cm or 0 cm.

### 2.5.2    Stadiometer

■    Follow the same procedures as for start of stand. Place the calibration on the floor of the stadiometer.

■    Place the horizontal bar of the stadiometer firmly against the top of the calibration rod. The digital display should read 80 cm.

■    Capture the counter reading in the QC Checks Weekly dialog box. Click the Done box corresponding to the stadiometer when the calibration is complete. If the stadiometer display does not read 80cm, you will need to recalibrate it.

■    To recalibrate, adjust the stadiometer headpiece digital display to read 80 cm by pressing the + or − button. Note in the comment box that the stadiometer was recalibrated.

### 2.5.3    Skinfold Calipers

■    Follow the same procedures as for start of stand. Zero the calipers before starting the calibration procedures. Place the step wedge standard between the caliper arms at each of the four steps, and check that the reading falls within the acceptable range.

■    Record the measurement taken at each step in the QC Checks Weekly dialog box Result field. Click the Done box corresponding to the skinfold calipers when the calibration is complete. An identical calibration should be done on the spare set of skinfold calipers and the corresponding measurements also recorded in the QC Checks dialog box.

- If the caliper readings fall outside the acceptable range at any level, use the other set of calipers and inform the MEC manager. They will be returned to the manufacturer for adjustment.

- If the calipers become too loose, use the spare set of calipers and inform the MEC manager.

- The acceptable ranges for the step wedge readings are as follows:

| | | | |
|---|---|---|---|
| first step | 9.8 – 10.5 | third step | 29.9 – 30.5 |
| second step | 19.8 – 20.5 | fourth step | 39.8 – 40.4 |

## 2.6    Daily Calibration Procedures

The scale is the only piece of equipment that will need to be calibrated daily.

### 2.6.1    Digital Weight Scale

- The scale is a fairly rugged piece of equipment that does not need frequent formal calibrations. However, to ensure it is functioning properly, you must do a "rough" calibration daily. First, step on the scale and weigh yourself, noting your weight. Second, add one or two 10-pound calibrated weights and check to make sure the displayed weight increases accordingly. Then capture this in the QC Checks Daily dialog box.

- If there is any reason to believe that the scale is not accurate, contact the MEC manager. The scale will need to be recalibrated by the service representative.

## 2.7    Care and Maintenance

To ensure the equipment functions properly and is hygienic, it must be maintained on a regular basis.

### 2.7.1    Cleaning Equipment

- At the beginning of each stand, and at the end of each examining day, wipe the surfaces of the sliding calipers, skinfold calipers, and tape measures with alcohol.

- Clean the stadiometer and infantometer aluminum track daily with a damp cloth.

- Lubricate the stadiometer and infantometer aluminum track as needed with CRC 3-36. Do this only at the _end_ of an examination day.

- Clean the acrylic parts of the stadiometer and infantometer with antistatic plastic cleaner.

- Clean the digital displays with a dry cotton cloth. Do not allow any fluids to drip into the display housing.

### 2.7.1.1    Maintenance for the Infantometer

- Each day check that the footboard moves up and down the track smoothly. If not, apply a small amount of lubrication (see Cleaning Equipment, Section 2.7.1). If the operation is still not smooth, inform the MEC manager.

### 2.7.1.2    Maintenance for the Stadiometer

- Each day check that the upright Plexiglas bar moves up and down the track smoothly.

- Check that the horizontal bar is firmly attached to the upright sliding section and that the section operates smoothly. If it does not, clean the upright bar with a damp cloth and lubricate the track with CRC 3-36 at the end of the day.

### 2.7.1.3    Maintenance for the Skinfold Calipers

"Zero" the calipers each time you take a measure. Check to make sure the pointer is clearly reading zero. If not, loosen the flat screw on top of the dial, turn the dial slowly and gently until the pointer reads zero and then turn the screw tight again.

### 2.7.2    Malfunctions

Report any malfunctions of the body measurement equipment to the MEC manager. Back-up equipment is provided in each MEC to be used until malfunctioning equipment can be repaired or replaced.

## 2.8    End of Stand Procedures

At the end of each stand, it is the responsibility of the health technologists to prepare the body measurement room and equipment for moving. The following procedures are to be observed.

### 2.8.1    Calibration Procedures

You will need to calibrate the digital scale before preparing it for travel. Follow the same procedures you used for the Start of Stand and Mid-Stand Calibration.

- Place all six of the 50-pound calibrated weights on the scale and capture the weight in the QC Checks dialog box, Start of Stand tab. Click the Done box corresponding to the scale when the calibration is complete.

- If there is any reason to believe that the scale is not accurate, notify the MEC manager to have the scale recalibrated by a service representative.

### 2.8.2    Pack-Up Procedures

You will need to pack-up all the supplies and equipment before closing up the MEC. Remove the supplies (e.g., alcohol, gauze pads, cosmetic pencils) and equipment (e.g., small sliding calipers, skinfold calipers, head circumference tape) from the baskets and put them in the drawers. Discard any leftover CRC 3-36; leaving it in the MEC or in a vehicle can be a fire hazard.

Additional procedures are needed for the calipers, scale, stadiometer, infantometer, and measurement box. These are described below.

### 2.8.2.1    Calipers

- Place the mediform calipers in the protective cases; store them in the third drawer of the cabinet.

- Place the skinfold calipers in the protective cases; store them in the third drawer of the cabinet.

### 2.8.2.2    Digital Weight Scale

- Place the cover on the scale.

- Put the seat above the scale down.


### 2.8.2.3    Stadiometer

- Push the headpiece to the bottom of the measurement column.

- Check to ensure that the screws at the top of the measurement column are in place. If necessary, tighten by giving them a few turns.


### 2.8.2.4    Infantometer

- Push the footpiece to the far left side of the infantometer.

- Place the strap around the metal base of the footpiece and attach the ends of the strap to the hooks on the wall.

- Wrap the bar code wand in padding and place between the footpiece and the end of the infantometer.


### 2.8.2.5    Measurement Box

- Push the box up against the stadiometer with the square piece of foam padding separating the two pieces of equipment. Secure the box by placing the strap around two legs of the box and attaching each end of the strap to a hook on the wall.


### 2.8.2.6    Body Measurement Cabinet

- All the equipment and supplies will be placed in the body measures cabinet for storage between stands. Each piece of equipment and all supplies will have a designated and labeled space for storage.

- Discard the plastic trash bag hung under the desk.

# 3. EXAMINATION PROTOCOL

## 3.1 Eligibility Criteria

All SPs are eligible for the body measurement component. Specific measurements are completed dependent on the age of the SP. Table 3-1 lists the SP age groups and the corresponding measurements, in the sequence they will be measured.

SPs aged 6+ are also eligible for the Physical Activity Monitor (PAM) component, to be conducted in the same examination room following body measurements (refer to Chapter 6, Physical Activity Monitor).

## 3.2 Pre-examination Procedures

Table 3-1. Body measurements, by age

| Birth+ | 2mo+ | 2yr+ | 4yr+ | 8yr+ |
|---|---|---|---|---|
| Weight | Weight | Weight | Weight | Weight |
| Recumbent length | Recumbent length | Recumbent length (through 47mos) | | |
| Head circumference | Head circumference **(through 6 mo.)** | | | |
| | | Standing height | Standing height | Standing height |
| | | | | Upper leg length |
| | | | | Maximal calf circumference |
| | Upper arm length | Upper arm length | Upper arm length | Upper arm length |
| | Arm circumference | Arm circumference | Arm circumference | Arm circumference |
| | | Waist circumference | Waist circumference | Waist circumference |
| | | | | Thigh circumference |
| | Triceps skinfold | Triceps skinfold | Triceps skinfold | Triceps skinfold |
| | Subscapular skinfold | Subscapular skinfold | Subscapular skinfold | Subscapular skinfold |

### 3.2.1　Measuring and Recording Guidelines

Body measurements are always taken on the right side of the body unless the SP has a cast, amputation, or for some other reason the measurement cannot be taken on the right side. When this occurs, take the measurement on the left side of the body.

All measurements, except skinfolds, should be taken to the nearest tenth of a centimeter or 1.0 millimeter. Skinfold measurements are taken to the nearest 0.1 millimeter. The computer will alert the recorder to all measures that are less than the 1st percentile or greater than the 99th percentile. The examiner will verify the measurement before going to the next measure.

### 3.3　Examination Procedures

This section includes the protocol procedures and the examination screens. The protocol procedures explain in detail how to take the body measures. The examination screens illustrate how to enter the data and move through the screens.

### 3.3.1　Protocol Procedures

A total of 12 body measures will be collected in the Anthropometry examination. Depending on the SP's age, a minimum of 3 and a maximum of 10 measures will be taken.

### 3.3.1.1　Weight

The SP's weight will be taken on a Toledo digital scale. Weight will be measured in pounds and converted to kilograms in the automated system. Infants should wear only diapers and children and adults should wear only underwear, disposable paper gowns, and foam slippers. (Women should wear underpants only.) Infants and toddlers who can't stand unassisted will be weighed with an adult. Have the parent or technologist stand alone on the platform, tare the scale, and have the person on the scale hold the infant or toddler to obtain only the child's weight. Holding the child will provide greater security and reduce movement that might otherwise affect the accuracy of the measurement. Instruct older children and adults to stand still in the center of the scale platform facing the recorder, hands at side, and looking straight ahead. When the SP is properly positioned and the digital readout is stable, the recorder will click on the capture button on the screen. If the examinee weighs more than 440 pounds, use two Seca digital scales (located in the fourth drawer of the cabinet), have the SP stand with one foot on each scale, and add the weight on each scale to obtain an approximation of his or her weight. Enter this into the weight box of the screen. Do not weigh examinees in torso casts, but ask them to estimate their weight and then document this estimation in the comment section of the automated system. In the event of a power outage or if the scale is not functioning properly, use a Seca digital scale. Turn the scale on by pressing the "On" button, and have the SP stand on the scale as described above. Call the weight to the recorder, who will enter it into the weight box of the automated system.

### 3.3.1.2 Standing Height

Standing height is an assessment of maximum vertical size. Take this measure on all SPs 2 years and older, who are able to stand unassisted. Standing height is measured with a fixed stadiometer with a vertical backboard and a movable headboard. Have the SP move or remove hair ornaments, jewelry, buns, and braids from the top of the head in order to measure stature properly.

Have the SP stand on the floor (see Exhibit 3-1) with the heels of both feet together and the toes pointed slightly outward at approximately a 60° angle. Make sure the body weight is evenly distributed and both feet are flat on the floor. Check the position of the heels, the buttocks, shoulder blades, and the back of the head for contact with the vertical backboard. Depending on the overall body conformation of the individual, all points may not touch. In such case, make sure the SP's trunk is vertical above the waist, and the arms and shoulders are relaxed.

Align the head in the Frankfort horizontal plane. The head is in the Frankfort plane when the horizontal line from the ear canal to the lower border of the orbit of the eye is parallel to the floor and perpendicular to the vertical backboard. Many people will assume this position naturally, but for some it may be necessary to make a minor adjustment. If required, gently tilt the head up or down until proper alignment is achieved with eyes looking straight ahead. Lower the headboard and instruct the SP to take a deep breath and stand as tall as possible. A deep breath will allow the spine to straighten, yielding a more consistent and reproducible stature measurement. Position the headboard firmly on top of the head with sufficient pressure to compress the hair. When the SP is properly positioned, tell the recorder to "capture" the height. Hold the headpiece in position until the computer verifies the reading. Then have the SP relax and step away from the stadiometer. In the event of a power outage or if the stadiometer is not functioning properly, push the headpiece to the top of the measurement column and obtain the SP's height using the tape measure mounted on the right side of the measurement column. Call the height to the recorder, who will enter it in the height box of the automated system.

Some SPs may have conditions that interfere with the specific procedures for measuring stature. One of the more common conditions is kyphosis. Kyphosis is a forward curvature of the spine that appears as a hump or crooked back condition. Kyphosis most frequently occurs in the elderly, and in women the condition is commonly referred to as dowager's hump. In these cases it is important to get the best measurement possible according to the protocol. Then select the "NS" (not straight) comment.

Exhibit 3-1. SP position for standing height

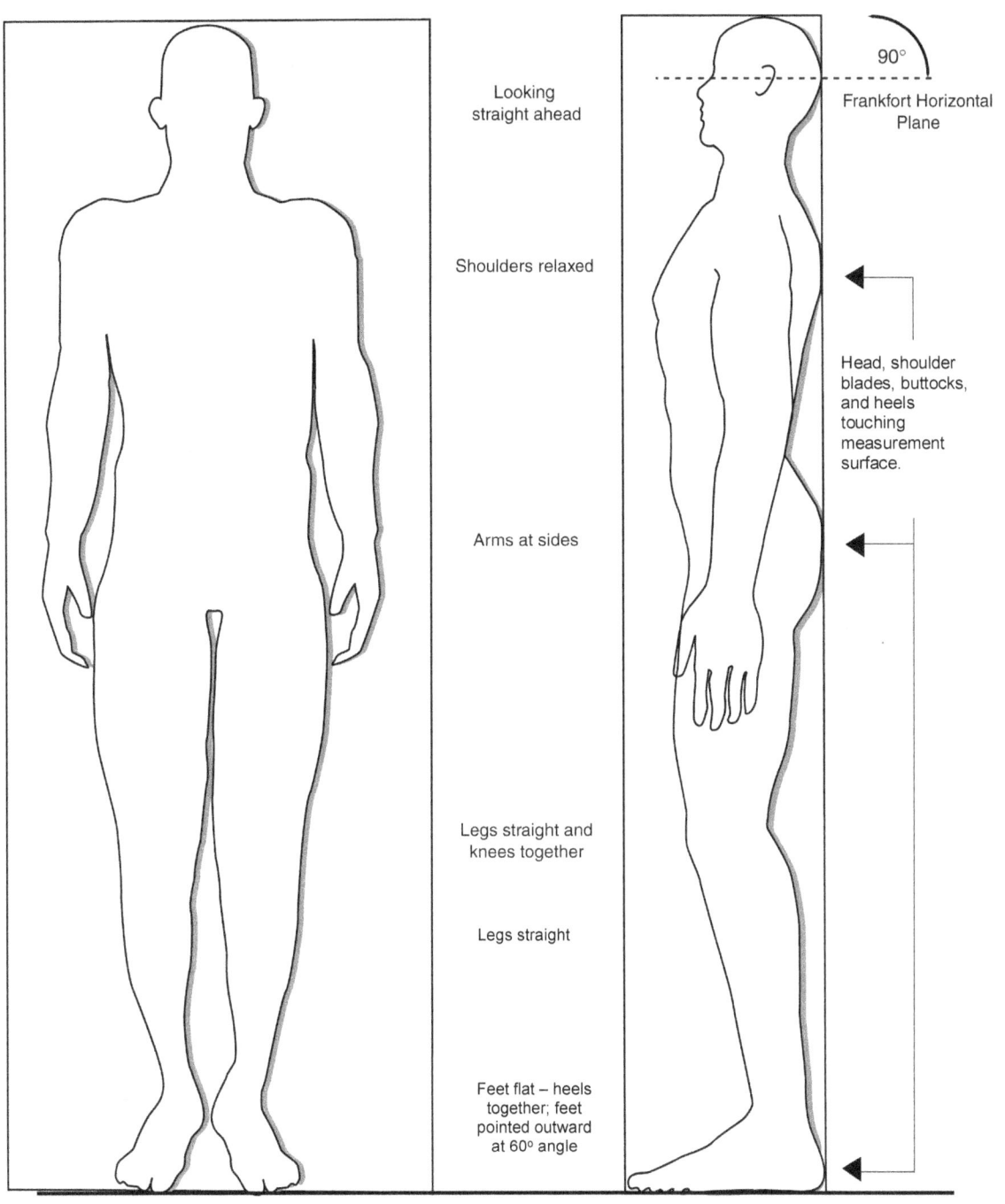

Looking
straight ahead

Shoulders relaxed

Arms at sides

Legs straight and
knees together

Legs straight

Feet flat – heels
together; feet
pointed outward
at 60° angle

90°

Frankfort Horizontal
Plane

Head, shoulder
blades, buttocks,
and heels
touching
measurement
surface.

### 3.3.1.3    Upper Leg Length

To reliably measure circumferences on the legs, the leg length must first be measured and the midpoint located and marked. The measuring box should be against the far wall near the exit door when the SP enters the room. Have the SP sit on the measuring box with the right knee bent at a 90° angle. Cut the right leg of the SP's exam pants up the leg so that the skin can be marked. Reassure the SP that the pant leg will be retaped after the body measurements are completed.

Position the small sliding caliper as if you were measuring the breadth of the patella. Position the caliper blades against the distal end of the femur on either side of the patella. The horizontal bar of the caliper should be touching, or close to the anterior surface of the thigh, proximal to the patella. Using the superior edge of the horizontal bar of the caliper as a guide, mark a line with a wax-based cosmetic pencil on the anterior surface of the thigh. Place the zero end of the steel measuring tape at the inguinal crease, just below the anterior superior iliac spine (this is easily located if the hips are in a sitting position). Do not apply pressure at the inguinal crease. However, folds of fat tissue may have to be lifted on some obese SPs to measure at the crease. Lift the exam gown and pull the pants slightly to smooth out gathers. Extend the tape down the anterior midline of the thigh to the mark that was previously made proximal to the patella (see Exhibit 3-2). To check for proper location of the zero end, firmly place the thumb over the measuring tape at the site and instruct the SP to raise the thigh slightly. Positioned correctly, a tightening of the muscle tendon will be clearly felt. Call the length of the upper leg to the recorder to the nearest 0.1 cm. The computer will divide this distance by two (which indicates the midpoint of the thigh) and will call out the midpoint. Make a mark on the skin at this midpoint before removing the measuring tape. Cross this mark (+) with another mark that should extend on a line between the anterior superior iliac spine and the middle of the patella. This point defines the point at which the mid-thigh circumference is measured. After measuring upper leg length, move the measuring box to the stadiometer, pushing it up against the measurement column. This will make more space available to take the remaining measurements.

Exhibit 3-2. SP position for upper leg length location and upper leg midpoint

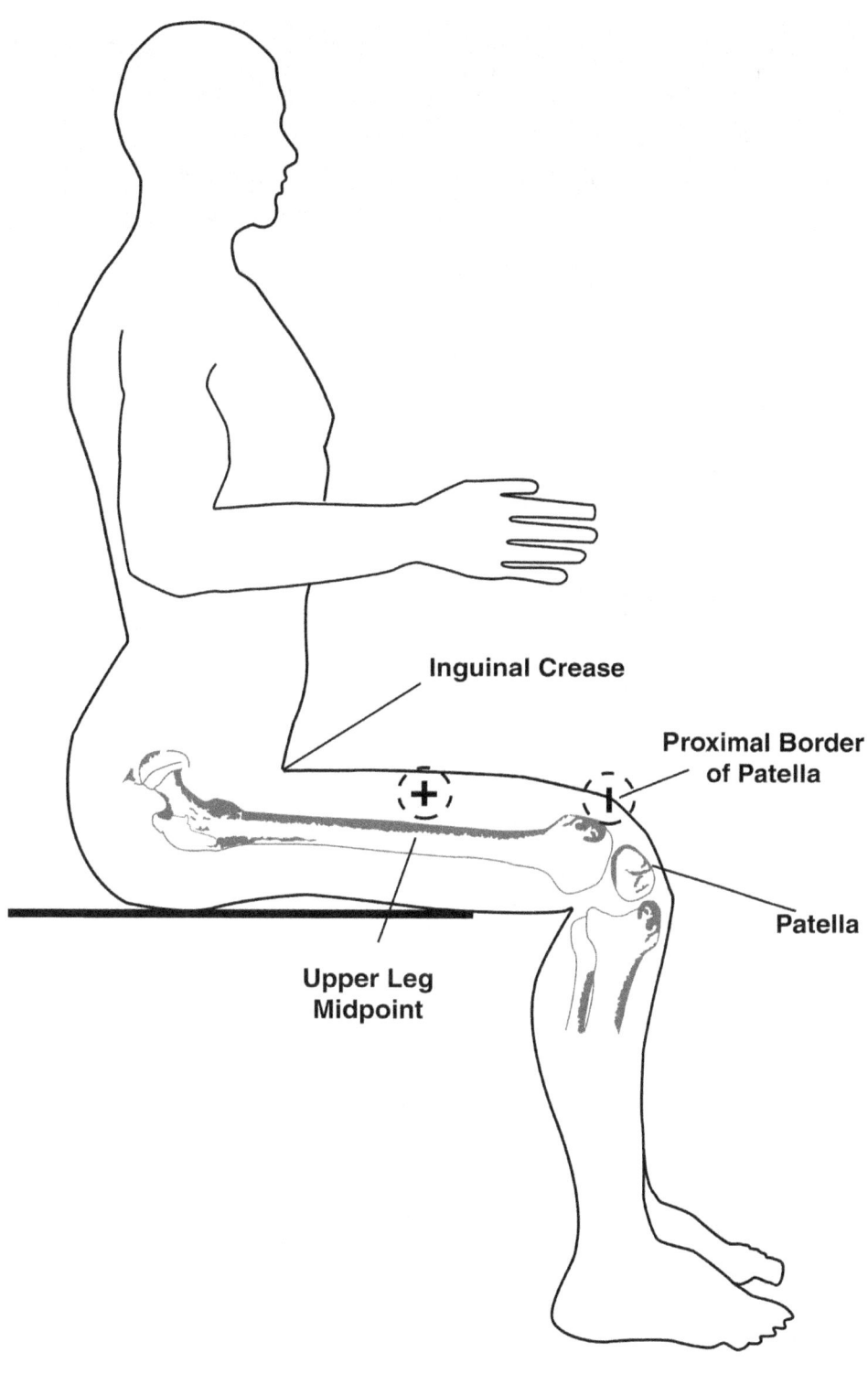

### 3.3.1.4 Maximal Calf Circumference

Measure the maximal calf circumference on the right calf (see Exhibit 3-3). While the SP is sitting, place the measuring tape around the calf and move it up and down to locate the maximum circumference in a plane perpendicular to the long axis of the calf. Hold the zero end of the tape below the measurement value, snugly but not tight. Call the calf circumference to the recorder to the nearest 0.1 cm. Ask the SP to stand, move away from the box, and turn toward the wall. Move the box to the base of the stadiometer. Then have the SP move toward the mirror, continuing to face the wall.

Exhibit 3-3. Measuring tape position for maximal calf circumference

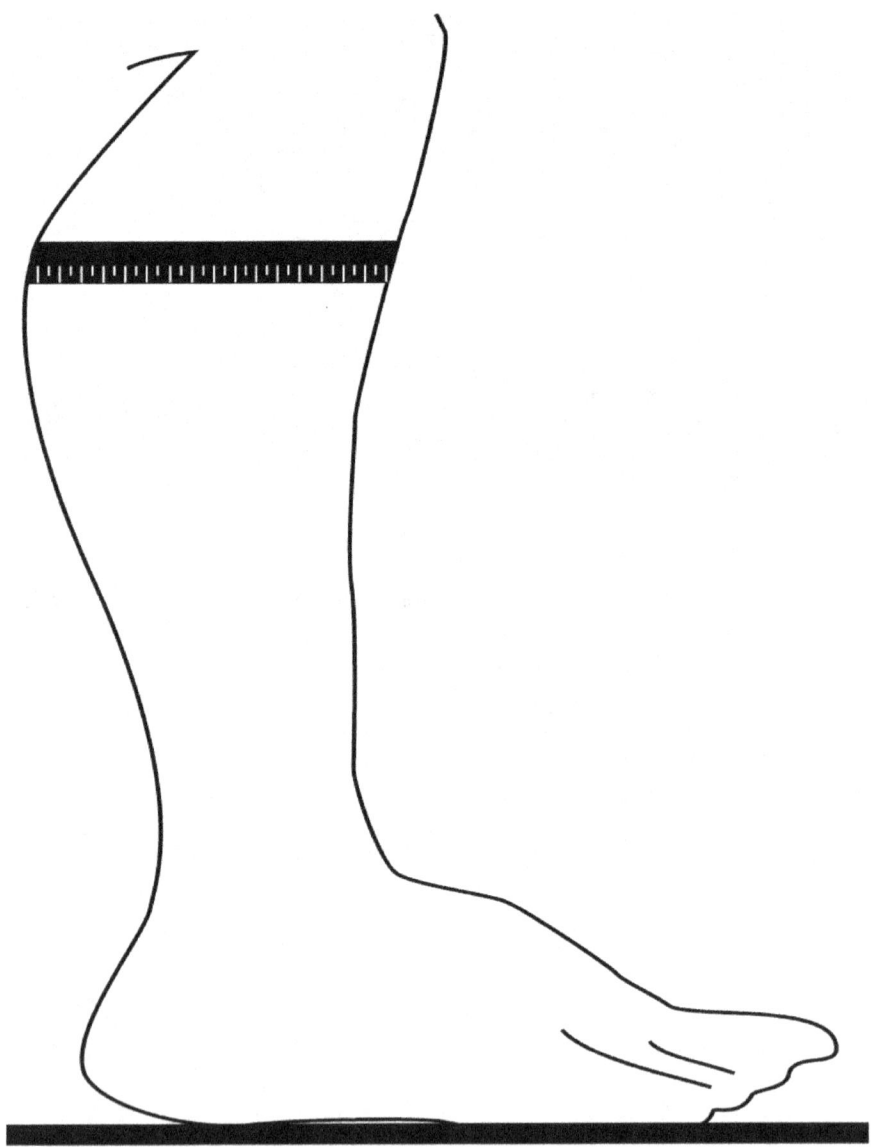

### 3.3.1.5      Upper Arm Length

To reliably measure circumferences and skinfolds on the arm, upper arm length must first be measured and the midpoint located and marked. Stand behind the SP to locate the middle of the upper arm. Have the SP stand erect with feet together and the right arm flexed 90° at the elbow with the palm facing up. On the right scapula, locate and <u>mark with a horizontal line</u> the uppermost edge of the <u>posterior</u> border of the acromion process (see Exhibit 3-4). This is also the best point at which to mark the inferior angle of the scapula in preparation for measuring the subscapular skinfold (see Section 3.3.1.9.2). Hold the zero end of the measuring tape at this mark and extend the tape down the posterior surface of the arm to the tip of the olecranon process (the bony part of the mid-elbow). Call the length of the upper arm to the recorder to the nearest 0.1 cm, keeping the tape in position. The computer will divide the distance by two and call out the midpoint. Make a horizontal mark with a cosmetic pencil at the midpoint at the posterior aspect of the arm. Cross this mark (+) with another mark that lies in a plane extending from the acromion to the olecranon process. This point defines the site at which both the midarm circumference and the triceps skinfold are measured.

### 3.3.1.6      Arm Circumference

Measure the arm circumference with the subject standing upright, shoulders relaxed, and the right arm hanging loosely. It is important to be certain that the muscle of the arm is not flexed or tightened, which could yield a larger and inaccurate reading. Stand facing the SP's right side and place the measuring tape around the upper arm at the crossed point (+), perpendicular to the long axis of the upper arm. Hold the measuring tape gently on the skin's surface. Pull the two ends of the overlapping tape together so that the zero end is held below the measurement value and the measurement is taken on the lateral aspect of the arm. Use care not to compress the skin and the underlying subcutaneous tissue. Call the arm circumference measurement to the recorder to the nearest 0.1 cm. Write the arm circumference on the gown for all SPs aged 8 years or older; this measurement will be used in the Physician component if the SP is sent to them after completing the Anthropometry component.

Exhibit 3-4. SP position for arm length and location of upper arm midpoint

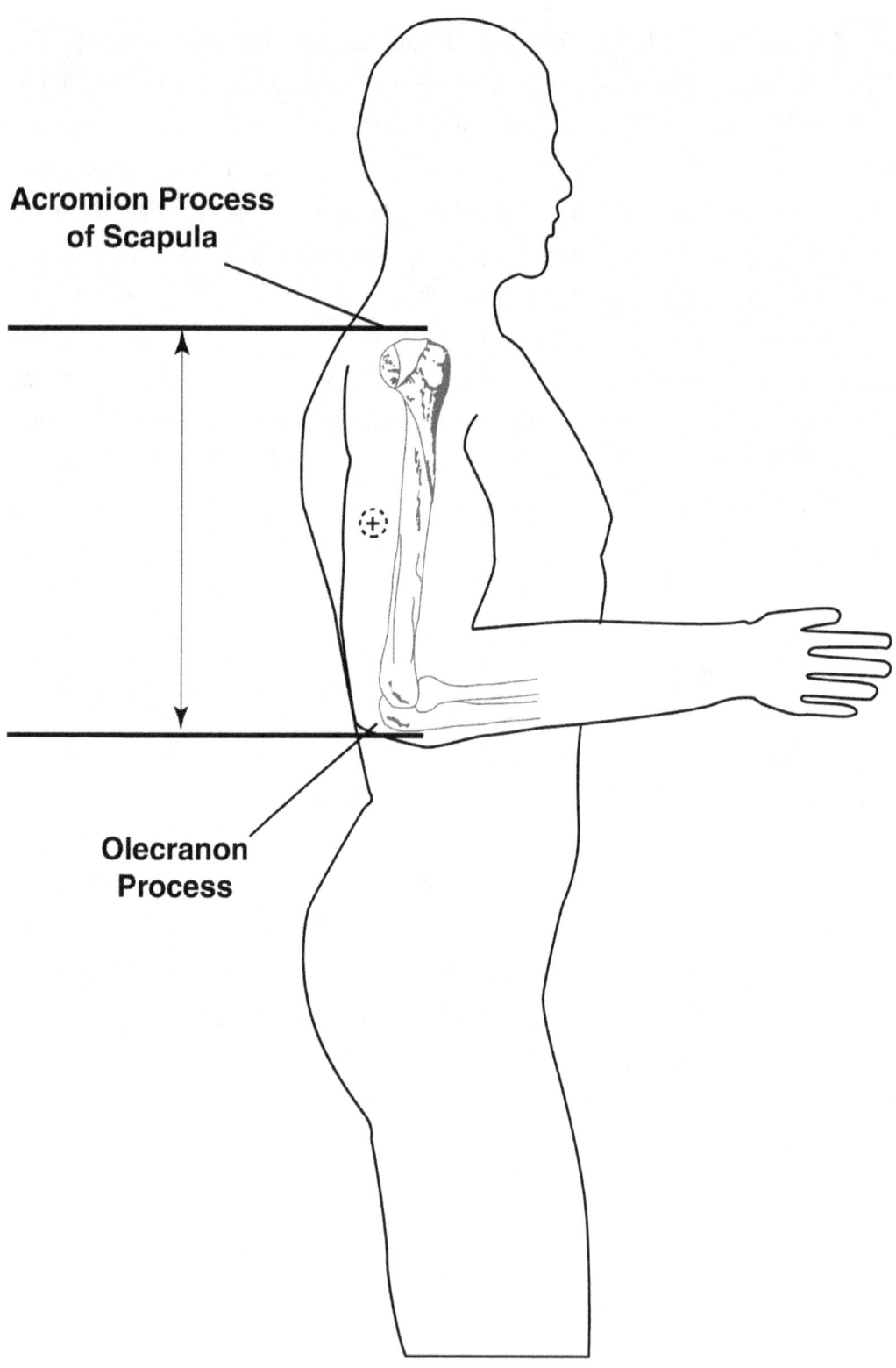

**Acromion Process
of Scapula**

**Olecranon
Process**

### 3.3.1.7    Abdominal (Waist) Circumference

To define the level at which the waist or abdominal circumference is measured, you must first locate and mark a bony landmark, the lateral border of the ilium. Have the SP stand and hold the examination gown above the waist. Lower the pants and underclothing of the SP slightly. Standing behind and to the right of the SP, palpate the hip area to locate the right ilium (see Exhibit 3-5). Draw a horizontal line just above the uppermost lateral border of the right ilium and then cross the line to indicate the midaxillary line of the body. Standing on the SP's right side, place the measuring tape around the trunk in a horizontal plane at the level marked on the right side of the trunk. Hold the zero end below the measurement value. Use the mirror on the wall to ensure correct horizontal alignment of the measuring tape. This is especially useful when measuring overweight SPs or women with hourglass-shaped torsos. The recorder should also observe the SP to make sure that the tape is parallel to the floor and that the tape is snug, but does not compress the skin. Make the measurement at the end of a normal expiration and call it to the recorder to the nearest 0.1 cm.

Exhibit 3-5. Measuring tape position for abdominal (waist) circumference

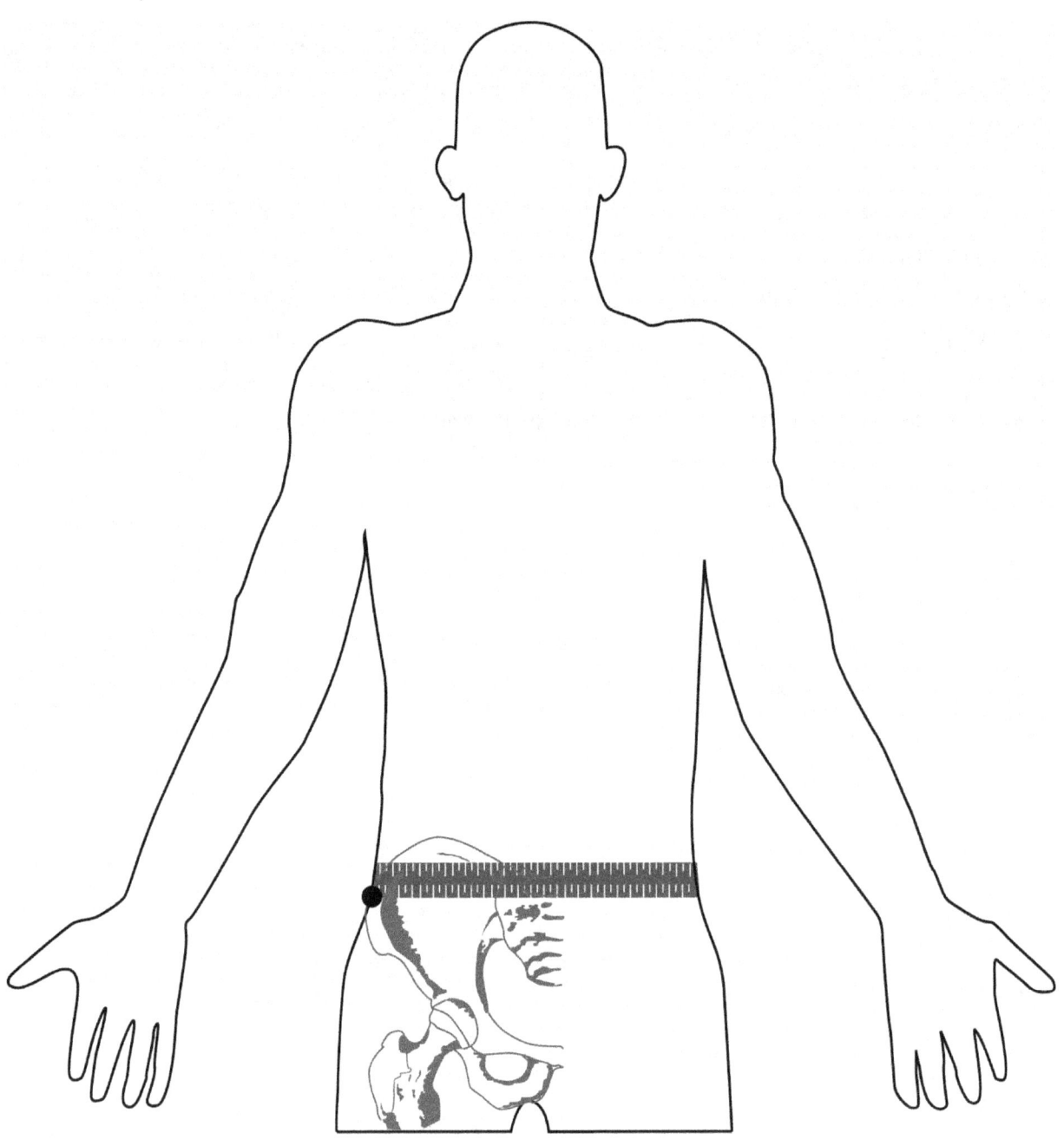

### 3.3.1.8    Thigh Circumference

For thigh circumference (see Exhibit 3-6), a standardized position is required. Explain this to the subject while demonstrating the position. Have the SP turn toward the recorder. Tell him or her to stand with most of the weight on the left leg with the right leg forward, knee slightly flexed, and soles of both feet flat on the floor. The bar on the exit door or the edge of the examining table may be used for the SP to hold onto to maintain balance. Stand on the SP's right side and place the measuring tape around the mid-thigh at the point that is already marked by a (+). Position the tape perpendicular to the long axis of the thigh with the zero end of the tape held below the measurement value. Rest the tape firmly on the skin but without compressing it. The recorder should check to make sure the tape is positioned correctly. Call the thigh circumference to the recorder to the nearest 0.1 cm.

Exhibit 3-6. Measuring tape position for thigh circumference

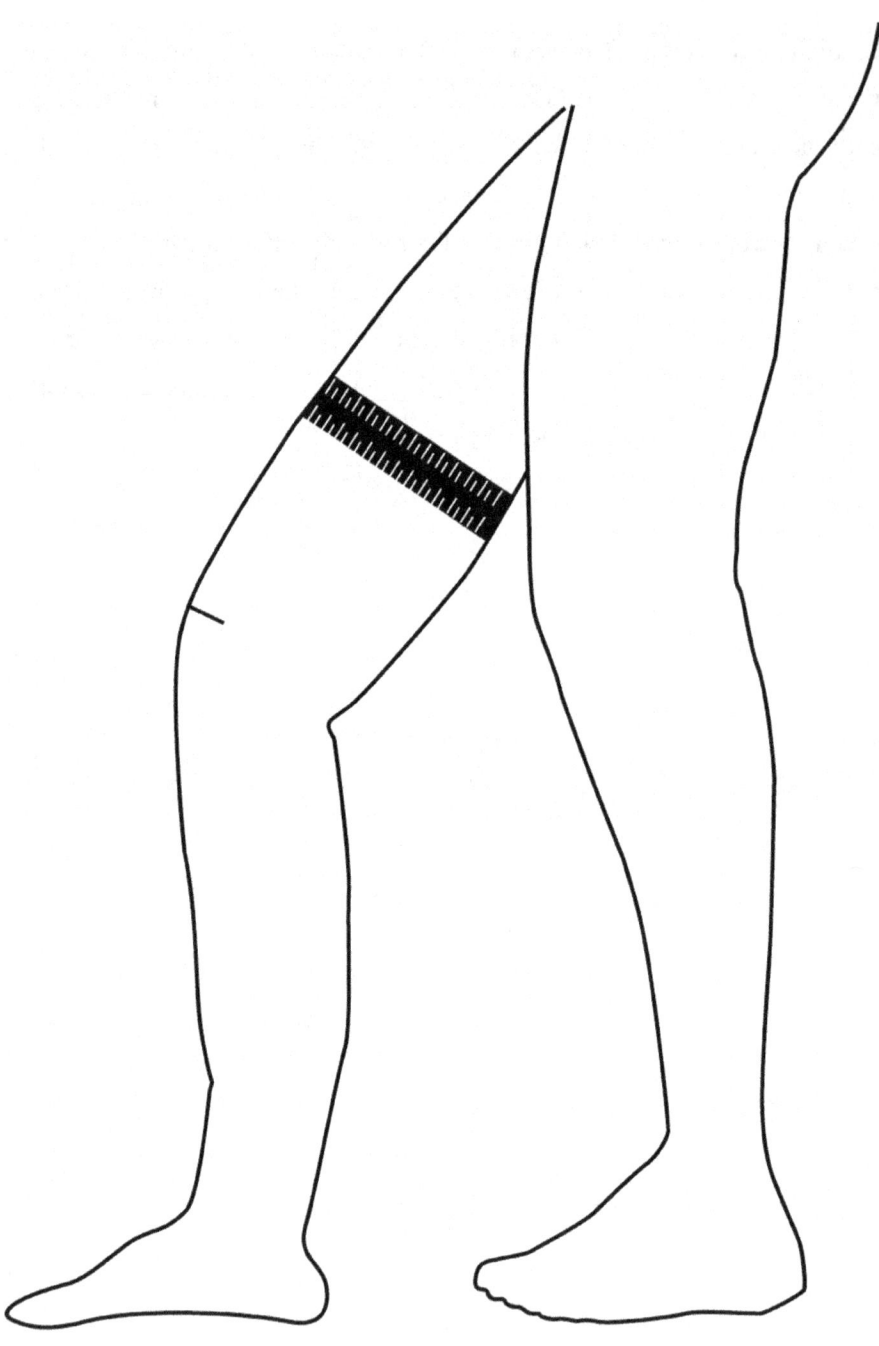

### 3.3.1.9    Skinfolds

Prior to measuring the skinfolds, you must mark each site carefully. Make all marks on the right side of the body. Use either a bony landmark on the trunk of the body or midpoints between two well defined bones on the limbs. In order to make young children comfortable with the measurement, explain the procedure and demonstrate the use of the caliper on the child's palm. Take all measurements with the Holtain skinfold calipers. Gently grasp the fold of skin and underlying subcutaneous adipose tissue between your left thumb and index finger. The amount grasped will depend upon the thickness of the subcutaneous adipose tissue. Grasp enough skin and adipose tissue to form a distinct fold that separates from the underlying muscle. The sides of the fold should be roughly parallel. The skinfold should be grasped 2.0 cm above the place the measurement is to be taken, and gently held with the thumb and forefinger. Place the jaws of the calipers <u>perpendicular</u> to the length of the fold. Exhibit 3-7 depicts both a double thickness of skin and underlying tissue, as well as the correct placement of the calipers for obtaining the measure. Measure the skinfold thickness to the nearest 0.1 mm while the fingers continue to hold the skinfold. Read the actual measurement from the caliper about 3 seconds after the caliper tension is released. Call the skinfold measurement to the recorder before releasing the fold. Remove the caliper, then release the fold of skin and subcutaneous fat. Record to the nearest 0.1 mm. The calipers can measure up to a maximum of 45 mm. When a distinct fold of skin and subcutaneous fat cannot be made with confidence (see Exhibit 3-8), enter the appropriate comment code that explains the situation.

## Exhibit 3-7 Diagram of a skinfold measurement

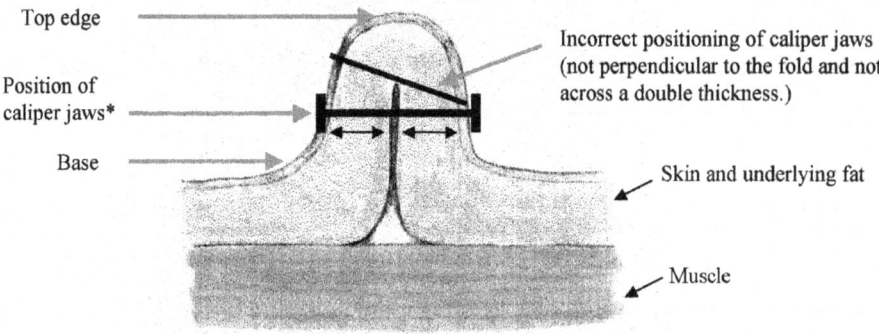

Double thickness of skin and underlying fat

Top edge

Position of caliper jaws*

Base

Incorrect positioning of caliper jaws (not perpendicular to the fold and not across a double thickness.)

Skin and underlying fat

Muscle

*Correct positioning of caliper jaws - perpendicular to the skinfold and across two thicknesses of skin and underlying fat.

## Exhibit 3-8. **Incorrect** measurement of a skinfold

Single thickness of skin and underlying fat

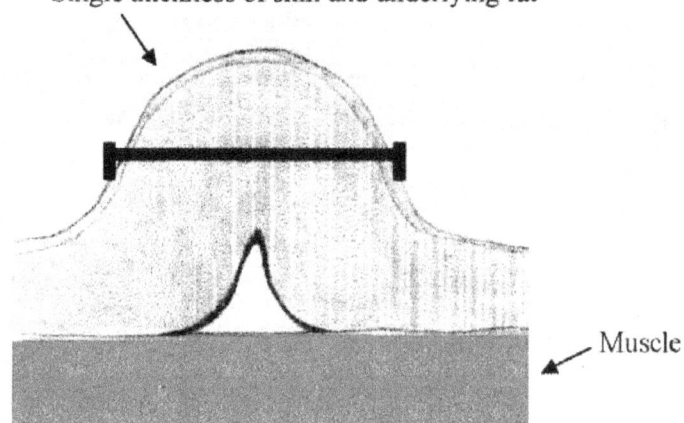

Muscle

### 3.3.1.9.1     Triceps Skinfold

Measure the triceps skinfold on the posterior surface of the right upper arm, at the point previously marked for the mid-upper arm circumference. Have the SP stand upright with weight evenly distributed and feet together, shoulders relaxed, and the arms hanging freely at the sides. Stand <u>behind</u> the SP's right side and gently grasp a fold of skin and subcutaneous adipose tissue with thumb and index finger, approximately 2.0 cm above the marked point. The skinfold should be <u>parallel</u> to the long axis of the arm (see Exhibit 3-9). Place the tips of the caliper jaws over the marked point, <u>perpendicular</u> to the length of the fold (see Exhibit 3-10). Measure the skinfold thickness to the nearest 0.1 mm while the fingers continue to hold the skinfold. Call the measurement to the recorder before releasing the fold and the caliper.

Exhibit 3-9. Location of triceps skinfold

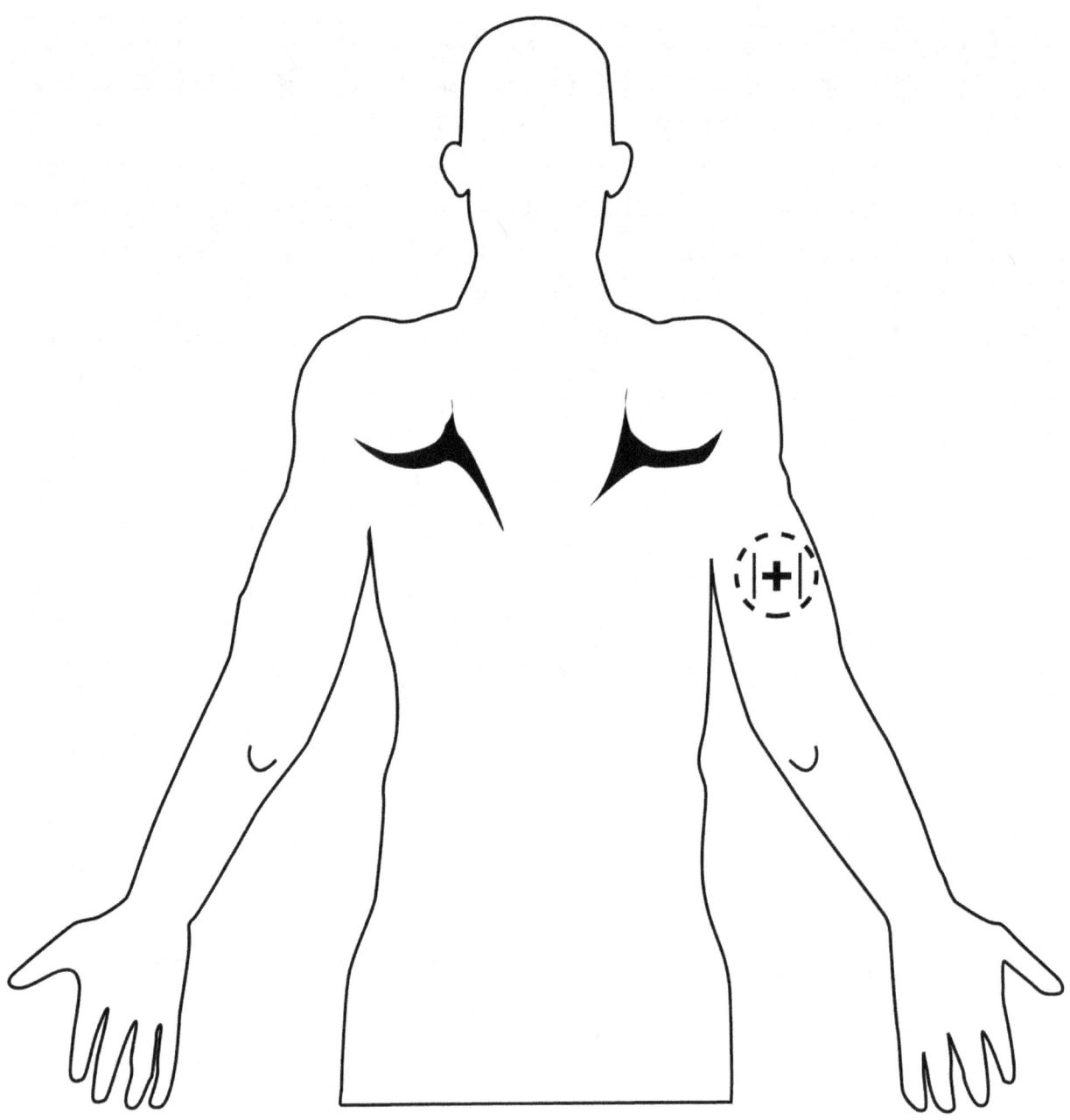

Exhibit 3-10  Correct placement of caliper jaws (triceps skinfold)

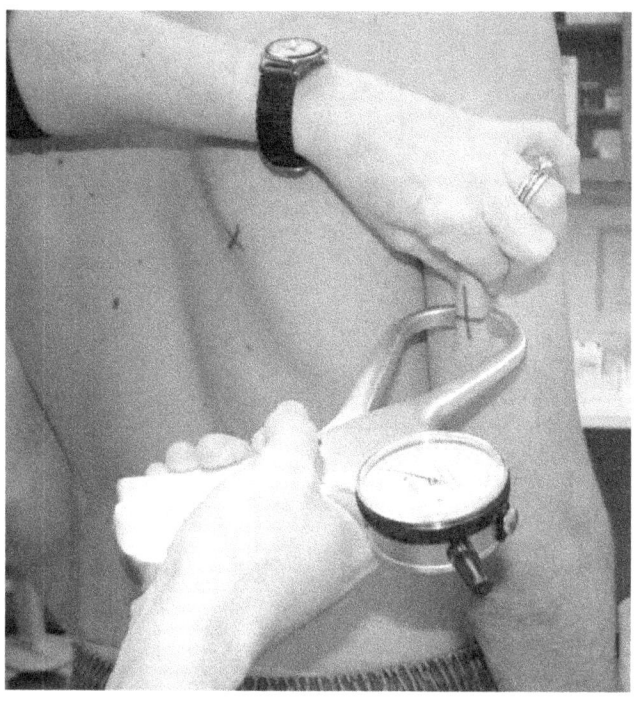

### 3.3.1.9.2    Subscapular Skinfold

Measure the subscapular skinfold with the SP standing erect with shoulders relaxed and arms hanging loosely at the side. Open the back of the examination gown and palpate for the inferior angle (or triangle portion) of the right scapula. Make a cross (+) <u>on</u> the inferior angle of the scapula with the cosmetic pencil marker. (The measures flow more smoothly if this mark is done after marking the acromium process of the scapula, prior to measuring upper arm length.) (See Exhibit 3-11 on page 3-20.) Gently grasp a fold of skin and subcutaneous adipose tissue with the index finger directly above (1.0 cm) and medial to the inferior angle of the scapula, with the thumb reaching toward the spine. The skinfold should form a line about 45 degrees below the horizontal extending diagonally toward the right elbow (see Exhibit 3-12). Place the tips of the caliper jaws perpendicular to the length of the fold about 2.0 cm lateral to the fingers with the top jaw of the caliper on the mark over the inferior angle of the scapula (see Exhibit 3-13). Measure the skinfold thickness to the nearest 0.1 mm while the fingers continue to hold the skinfold. Call the measurement to the recorder before releasing the fold and the caliper.

Exhibit 3-11. Location of subscapular skinfold

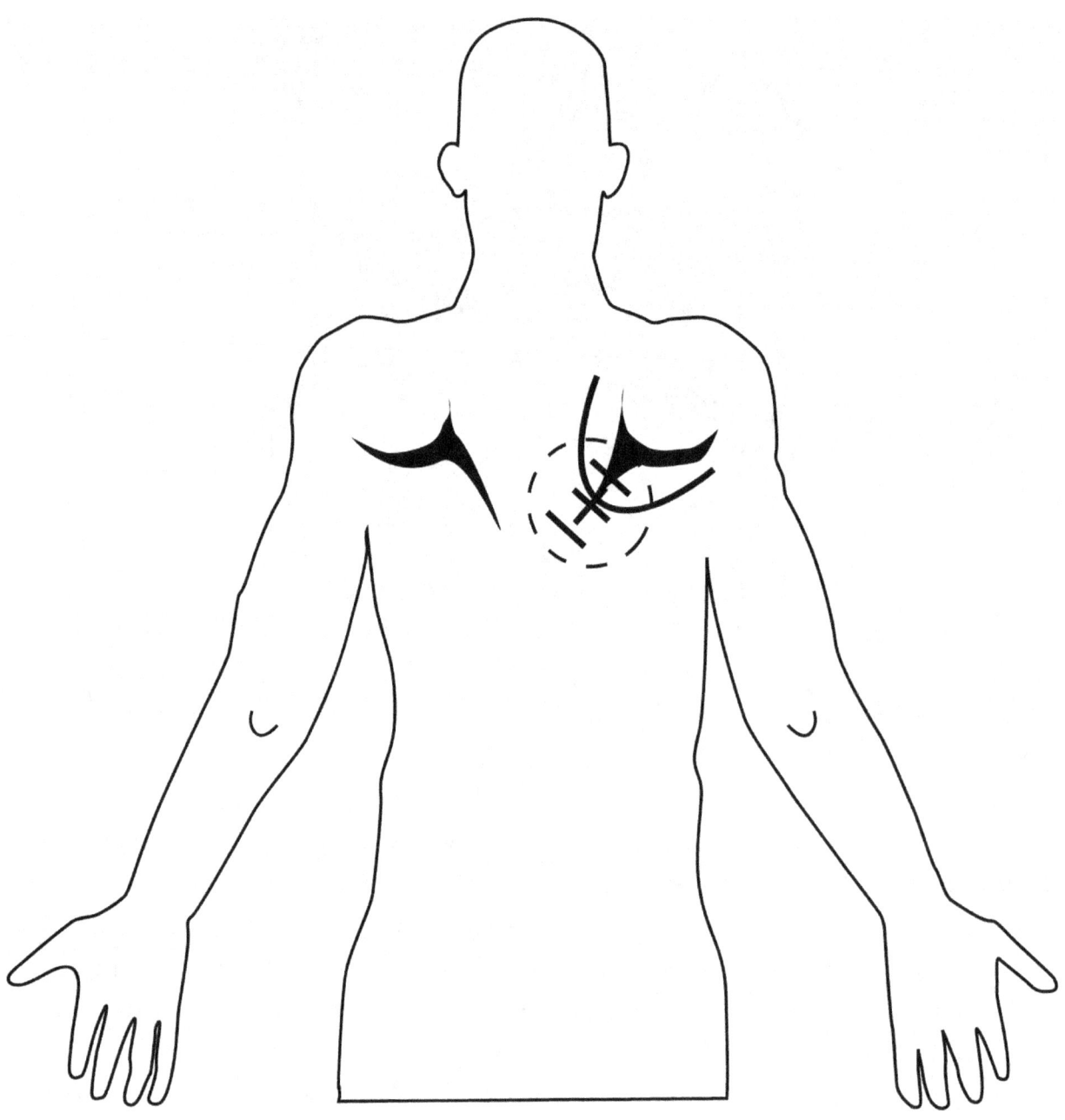

Exhibit 3-12  Proper grasping technique for subscapular skinfold

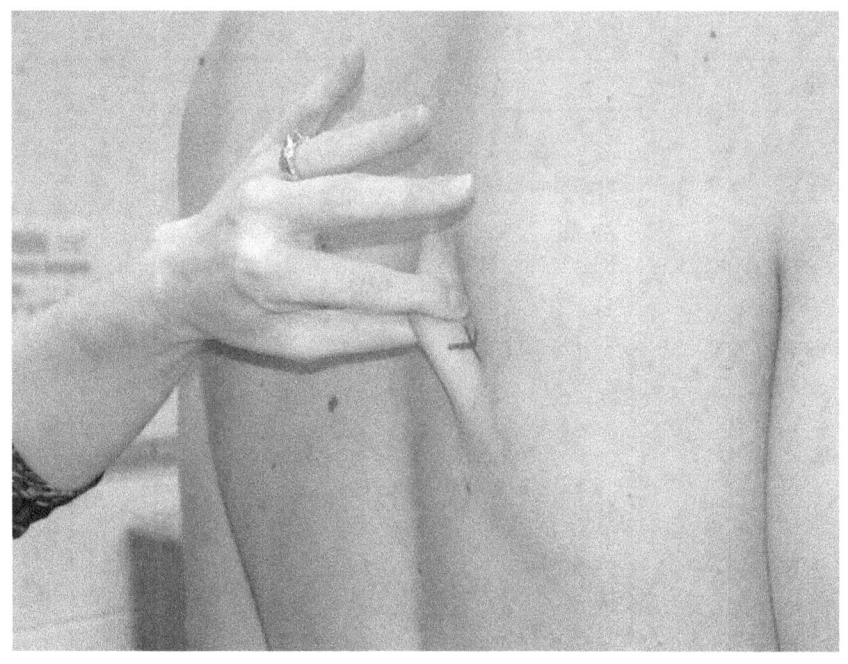

Exhibit 3-13  Correct placement of caliper jaws (subscapular skinfold)

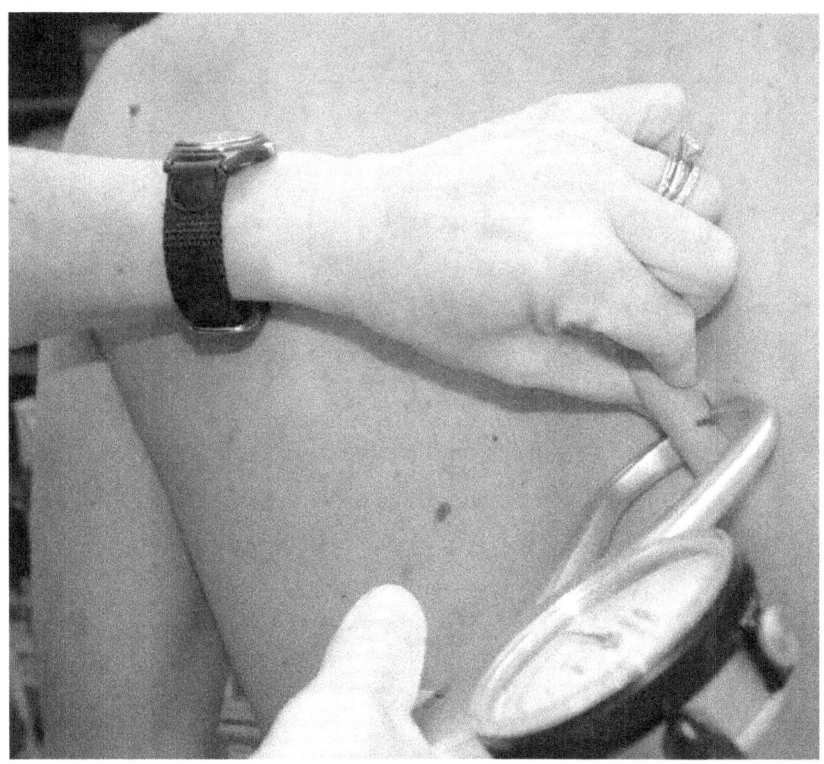

### 3.3.1.10 Sequence of Measurement Components, SP Position, and Examiner Equipment for SPs 4+

| Measurement | SP Position | Equipment |
|---|---|---|
| 1. Weight | Standing | Scale |
| 2. Standing height | Standing | Stadiometer |
| 3. Upper leg length (mid-mark is placed on SP) (8 + only) | Sitting on box <br> Right pant leg open | Small sliding caliper <br> Cosmetic pencil <br> Measurement box |
| 4. Maximal calf circumference (8+ only) | Sitting on box | Steel tape |
| 5. Upper arm length (mid-mark is placed on SP) | Standing | Steel tape <br> Cosmetic pencil |
| 6. Arm circumference | Standing | Steel tape |
| 7. Waist circumference (mark iliac crest) | Standing <br> Hold gown up | Steel tape <br> Cosmetic pencil |
| 8. Thigh circumference (8+ only) | Gather side seams of exam pants <br><br> Standing <br> Hold gown up <br> Right pant leg open | Steel tape |
| 9. Triceps skinfold | Standing | Skinfold calipers |
| 10. Subscapular skinfold | Standing | Skinfold calipers |

### 3.3.1.11 Measuring Children under 8 Years of Age

The same procedures are followed for measuring stature and weight of children aged 2 through 7 years, as used for older SPs. For measuring circumferences or skinfolds, the child may stand on the measuring box to allow the examiner to obtain measures at eye level. If the child is going to stand on the box, move it toward the mirror so that the child can hold onto the bar on the wall for support. If the child is too young to sit or stand by him or herself, take the measurements with the child sitting in the parent's lap. The examiner's eyes must be level with the calipers to prevent parallax. Otherwise, use the same procedures as with older SPs.

### 3.3.1.11.1 Recumbent Length

Recumbent length is measured on children less than 4 years of age (birth to 47 months). An Infantometer is used to take the measure. The measuring board has a fixed headpiece, a horizontal back piece, and a movable foot piece. Placing infants and small children in a recumbent position frequently generates a sense of insecurity and consequently invokes a crying response. When measuring recumbent length the parent or other caretaker of the child should be positioned between the examiner and recorder. The parent should encourage and comfort the child by making eye contact, talking to, and if necessary, holding the head of a restless child. The recorder supports the child's head. Similar to the procedure with standing height, the child's head is positioned in the Frankfort plane. Gentle traction is applied to bring the top of the head in contact with the fixed headpiece. The child's head must be firmly held in this position by gently cupping the palms of the hands over the ears and holding the head in proper alignment. Simultaneously, the examiner aligns the child's legs by placing one hand gently but firmly over the knees. The toes point directly upward with the soles of the feet perpendicular to the horizontal backpiece of the measuring device. Gentle pressure is applied at the knees to keep the legs straight. The examiner then slides the movable foot piece to rest firmly at the child's heels. When the child is properly positioned, the recorder will click on the capture button on the screen. In the event of a power outage or if the infantometer is not functioning properly, the examiner will position the child as described above and read the length using the tape measure mounted on the board of the infantometer. The examiner will then call this measurement to the recorder, who will enter it in the recumbent length box.

### 3.3.1.11.2 Head Circumference

This measurement is done on children from birth through 6 months (see Exhibit 3-14). The child either sits in the parent's lap, on the footstool, or stands, depending upon age and activity level. The insertion tape is placed across the frontal bones just above the eyebrows, around the head above the ears on each side, and over the occipital prominence at the back of the head. The examiner holds the insertion tape snugly around the head. Hair ornaments and braids should be removed. The insertion tape is moved up and down over the back of the head to locate the maximal circumference of the head. The insertion tape should be perpendicular to the long axis of the face and should be pulled firmly to compress the hair and underlying soft tissues. Record the measurement to the nearest 0.1 cm.

Exhibit 3-14. Insertion tape position for head circumference

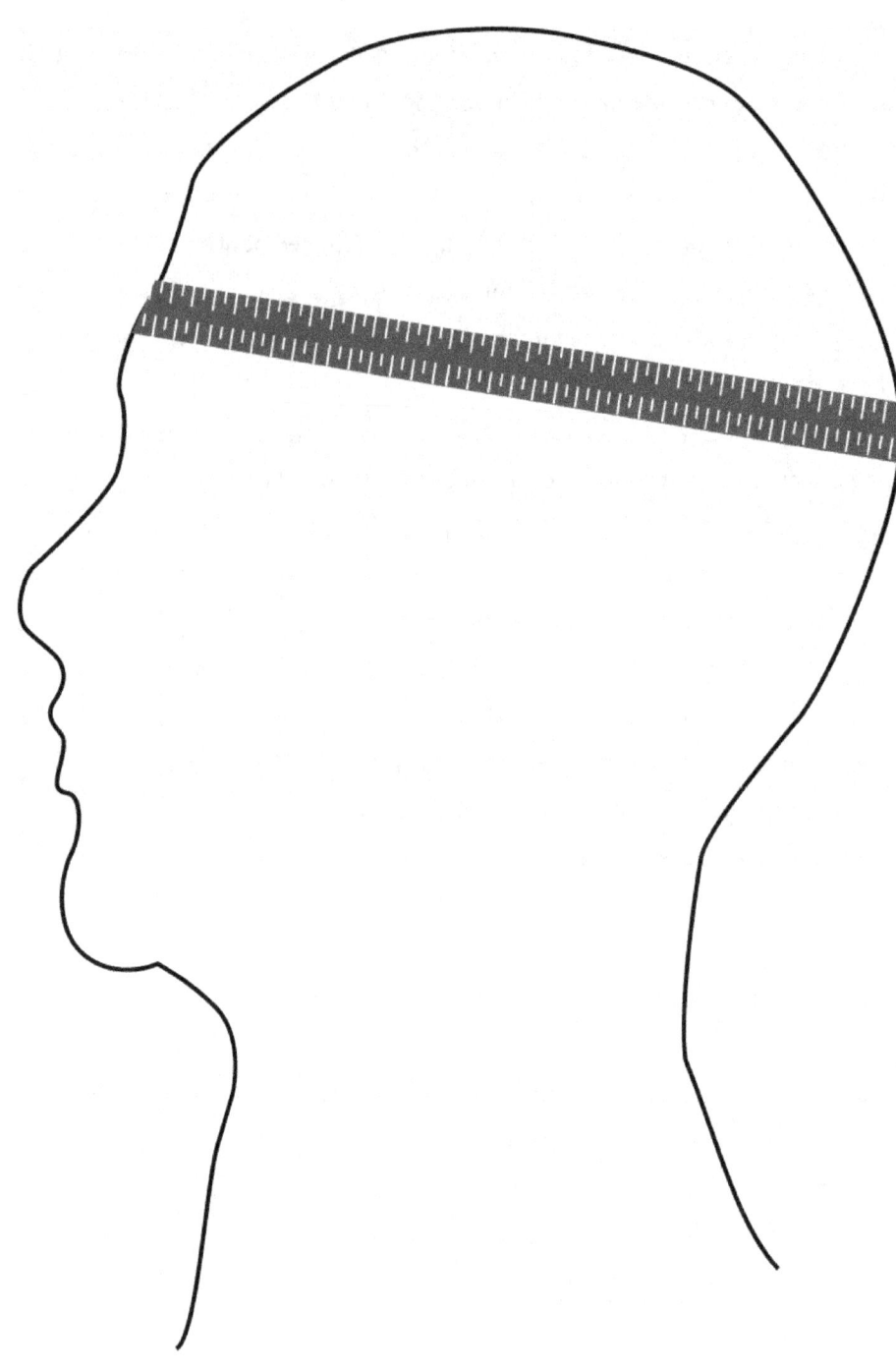

### 3.3.1.12    Measuring Handicapped SPs

Only limited anthropometric data can be collected on those SPs who are handicapped (in wheelchairs):

- Upper arm length is measured as if the SP was standing. It is necessary to position the SP over to the right side of the wheelchair so that the arm of the chair does not restrict the right arm.

- Arm circumference is also measured as if the SP was standing. The SP should be in the same position in the wheelchair as for measuring upper arm length. Again, it is important that the right arm is extended so that it is not restricted by the arm of the wheelchair.

- The triceps skinfold is measured on the back of the right arm as if the SP was standing. The position of the SP and the right arm are the same as for measuring arm circumference.

- Head circumference can be recorded in the same manner as an ambulatory child.

### 3.3.1.13    Measuring Amputees

Although the number of people with this condition will be small, for SPs who have any part of a limb on the right side amputated, the procedure is to collect the data on the SP's left side. This will, in most cases, eliminate the possibility of missing data (i.e., CNO [could not obtain]) for these situations.

For example, if the SP has any part of his/her right arm missing, you would do the Upper Arm Length measure, and mark the midpoint on the left arm. Additionally, you would measure the Arm Circumference and Triceps Skinfold on the left arm. If however, the SP has both arms missing, you would need to enter CNO in the Comment box for these three measures.

Be sure to enter this information accurately in the Amputations Screens before entering the status and finishing the exam. In these screens you will need to indicate the specific extremity(ies) that is missing. (See Section 3.3.2 and Exhibit 3-22.)

### 3.3.1.14    Tips for Anthropometry

### 3.3.1.14.1    General Comments

- Talk to the SP as you are moving through the measurements. Explain why and what you are doing, especially when locating the leg tendon in the groin area, and **before adjusting the pants down** to feel for the hip bone.

- Remain completely professional and unaffected by tattoos, body piercings, etc. DO NOT COMMENT about the SP's body.

- When you are taking the circumference and skinfold measurements, remember to stay in one place and move the SP around, rather than moving around the SP.

- If an SP has refused to change into an examination gown, complete as many measurements as possible. If the SP is wearing a loose fitting short sleeve or sleeveless shirt, it may be possible to obtain upper arm length, arm circumference and tricep skinfold measurements. Be sure to note 'CL' if an SP is wearing street clothes for a weight measurement.

### 3.3.1.14.2    General Comments for Children

- Unless they are too big, always place children 2-6 years old on the box so that you can control their movements and take the measurements at eye level. Be sure the box is moved toward the mirror so that the child can hold onto the bar on the wall for balance.

- For maximum control when measuring the arm circumference and skinfold of an infant, have the parent seated on the box with the infant situated over the left shoulder.

- When measuring the length of infants, make sure the head is in the Frankfort plane and that at least one leg is straight and the foot flexed. Remember, to get the child to flex his foot, run your fingernail down the inside of the foot.

- Make sure you have the mouse positioned on the 'GET' button before positioning the child, so that you can quickly capture the length. The only time you should enter the recumbent length manually is when you have no way of holding the child still while you capture the length.

- Do not let the calipers become the object of the child's attention. Keep them behind your body until you are ready to take the measure. It often helps to warm them up by holding them in your hand.

- If a child has not been changed into an examination gown, complete as many measurements as possible. Ask if the parent minds if an infant's clothes are removed, which would allow all measurements to be completed. If the infant's clothes are not removed, get all measurements possible. Be sure to note 'CL' if a child or infant is wearing street clothes for a weight measurement.

### 3.3.1.14.3   Standing Height

- Make sure the head and heels are against the stadiometer before taking the height, unless this position is anatomically impossible. DO NOT FORGET to have the SP take a deep breath and hold it while you position the headboard. If the SP is unable to stand with the head and heels against the stadiometer, make sure the trunk is vertical above the waist, and that the arms and shoulders are relaxed.

### 3.3.1.14.4   Upper Arm Length

- Position the SP's right arm so it is flexed 90° at the elbow with the palm facing up.

- Locate the acromium by following the scapula out to the arm until it makes a sharp turn to the front of the body. Draw the line on the bone before it turns to the front.

- Bring the tape measure out before bringing it down to ensure the tape is in the middle of the arm.

- Take the measure at the tip of the olecranon process (the bony part of the mid-elbow).

### 3.3.1.14.5   Maximal Calf Circumference

- Slide the tape measure up and down the calf to find the widest point. Take the measure there.

### 3.3.1.14.6   Skinfolds

- Take the measurements at eye level.

- If the triceps skinfold is hard to separate, start at the elbow (where the skin/fat is looser), and work up to the mark.

- If skinfolds are tight, take measure closer than ¾ inch to your fingers.

- For the subscapular skinfold, place the fingers ¾ inch above the X; only the top jaw of the caliper needs to be **ON** the X.

## 3.3.2    Examination Screens

Once the coordinator has assigned an SP to the body measures room, a communication dialog box from the coordinator will appear to let you know that an SP has been assigned to body measures. Click on the Close button to remove the dialog box from the screen.

Move the mouse pointer to the first icon on the left in the Standard toolbar. This is the "Logon SP" icon. Click on this button to begin the examination. A dialog box will appear, which will ask you for the *Examiner's* name and password. Wand the bar code on the SP's plastic bracelet to enter the ID. This will activate a dialog box containing descriptive information about the SP (i.e., name, SP ID, age, etc.). Confirm the name and check the age and sex to ensure you have the correct SP. Click OK to proceed with the examination.

### 3.3.2.1 General Screen Information

All screens have similar characteristics. As shown below, at the very top of the screen is a Title bar, with the component name (Anthropometry Subsystem), the Stand number, Session number, and the date and Session times. The Menu bar is just below the title bar, and the Standard toolbar icons are below the Menu bar. The Standard toolbar contains a row of buttons that provide shortcuts to menu commands as well as some other features. The Menu and Standard toolbars are described in the chapter on the MEC Automated System.

Just below the Standard toolbar is a second Title bar. This Title bar identifies the examination (Anthropometry Exam), the Stand number, Session number, and the Session's date and time. Below the Title bar is the SP ID, name, age, gender, and the current date and time. Below this bar, at the top left of the main area of the window, is the screen name.

Exhibit 3-15. Screen characteristics

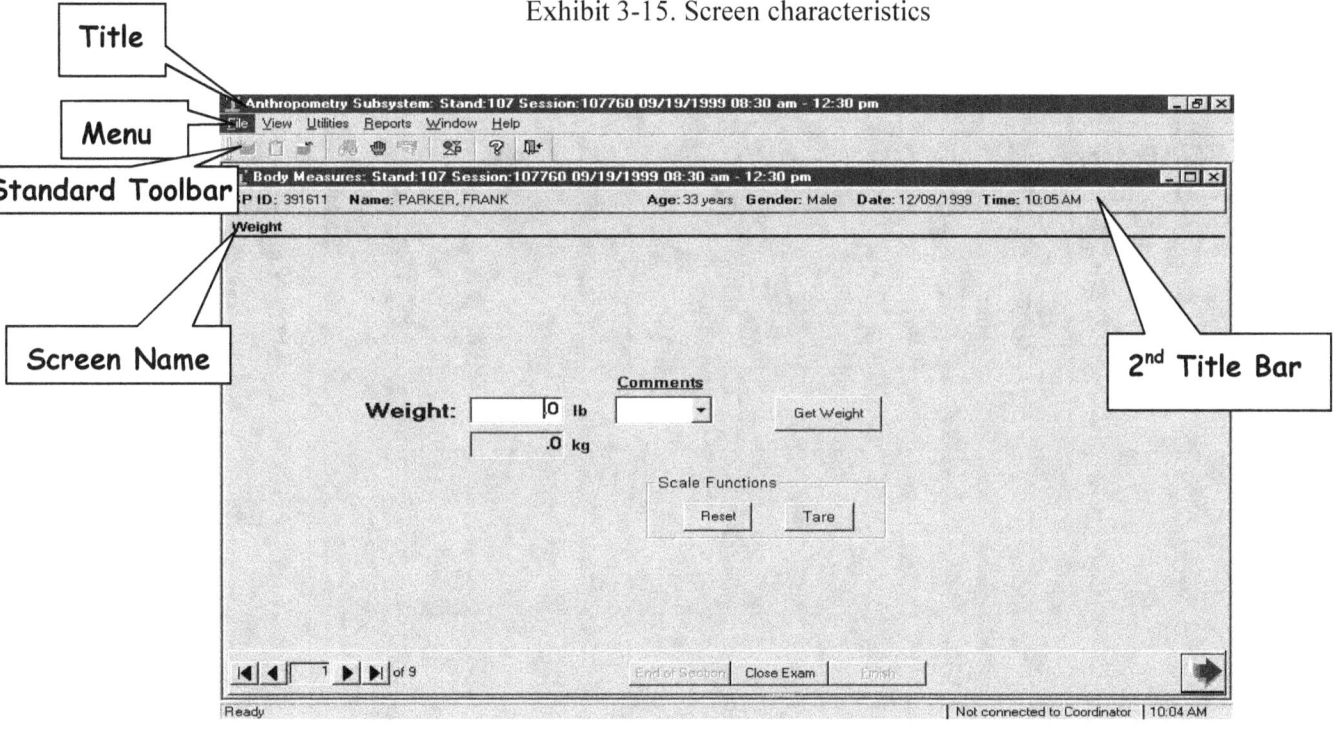

At the bottom left side of the screen is a screen number with a set of VCR arrow buttons on each side. These buttons help you navigate through the screens. The button on the far left moves you to the first screen. Likewise, the button on the far right moves you to the last screen. The button directly to the left of the screen number moves you to the previous screen, and the button directly to the right moves you to the next screen. Clicking on the arrow button will move you through the screens. At the bottom of the screen in the middle are two buttons, "Close" and "Finish," and to the far right is a large arrow. Clicking on the large arrow will move you to the next screen.

Exhibit 3-16. Navigation buttons

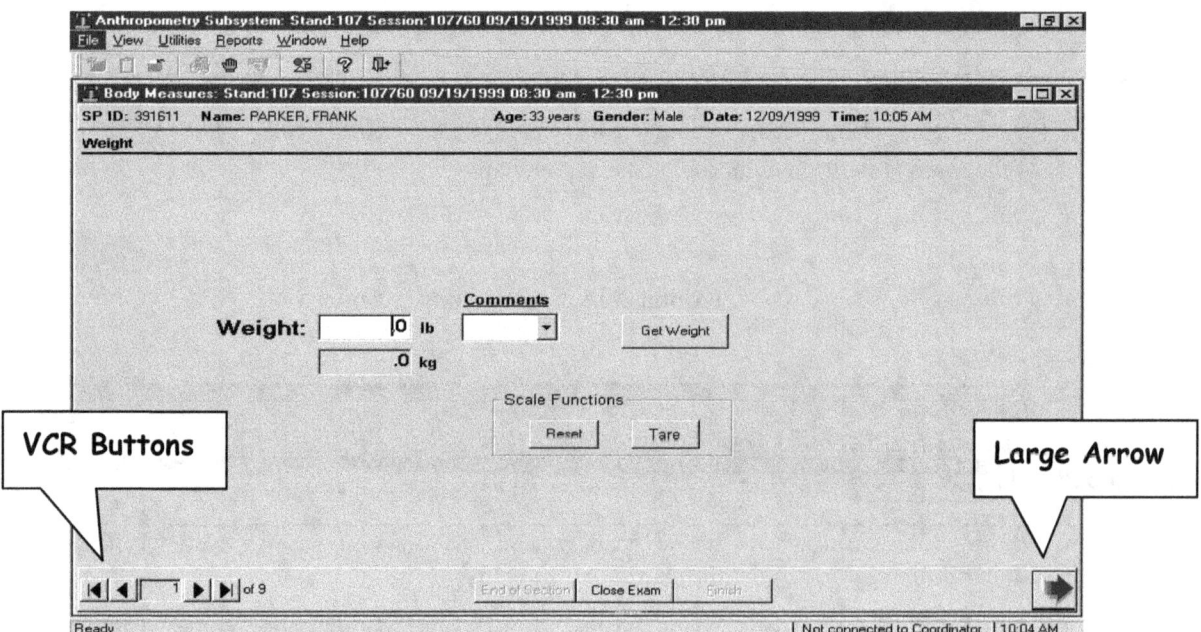

As you proceed through the examination entering data, you may activate an Edit Check box. This box will appear if you enter a measure in the system that is out of range (i.e., is less than the 1st or greater than the 99th percentile for the SP's age and sex). As shown below, the box reads "Check that measure." Read the box aloud to prompt the examiner to take another look at the measure.

Exhibit 3-17. Edit Check box

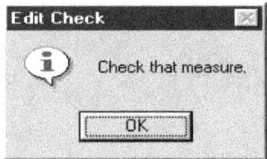

### 3.3.2.2    Weight Screen

The **Weight** screen is always the first data entry screen that will appear. Weight is collected on all SPs, regardless of age. The cursor will appear in the Weight field. After the SP steps on the scale, you will move the pointer to the "Get Weight" button, and click. The SP's weight is captured and displayed in the Weight field. If needed, you can select a comment by clicking on the down arrow to the right of the Comments box to activate a drop-down list. If a weight was not captured, you must enter either EC for "exceeds capacity" or CNO for "could not obtain." If the weight was captured, but the SP had on clothes rather than a gown, enter CL for "clothing." If the weight was captured but was inaccurate due to a medical appliance, such as a cast that could not be removed, enter MA for "medical appliance."

If an infant or toddler SP cannot be weighed unassisted, they will be weighed with an adult. The parent or examiner will stand alone on the scale platform while you click on the "Tare" button. Then the person on the scale will hold the SP while you move the pointer to the "Get Weight" button, and click. The system will capture the child's weight and display it on the screen. This procedure will assure that the weight is accurately collected. You will then move to the next screen by hitting "Enter" on the keyboard, or clicking on the large arrow in the lower right corner.

Exhibit 3-18. Weight screen

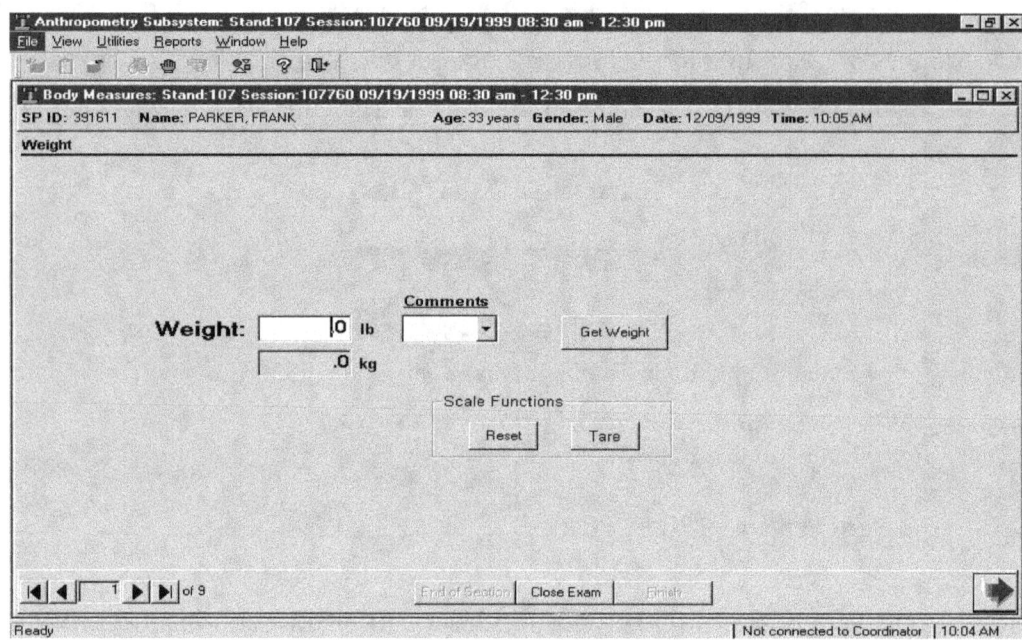

### 3.3.2.3    Stature Screen

The **Stature** screen is the second screen to appear. The measures on this screen are dependent on the age of the SP. The screen for SPs 0-6 months old will include Recumbent Length and Head Circumferences; the screen for SPs 7-23 months will only contain Recumbent Length; and the screen for SPs 24-47 months will include Recumbent Length as well as Standing Height. The stature screen displayed for all SPs 4 years of age or older includes Standing Height only.

Exhibit 3-19. Stature screens, depending on age of SP

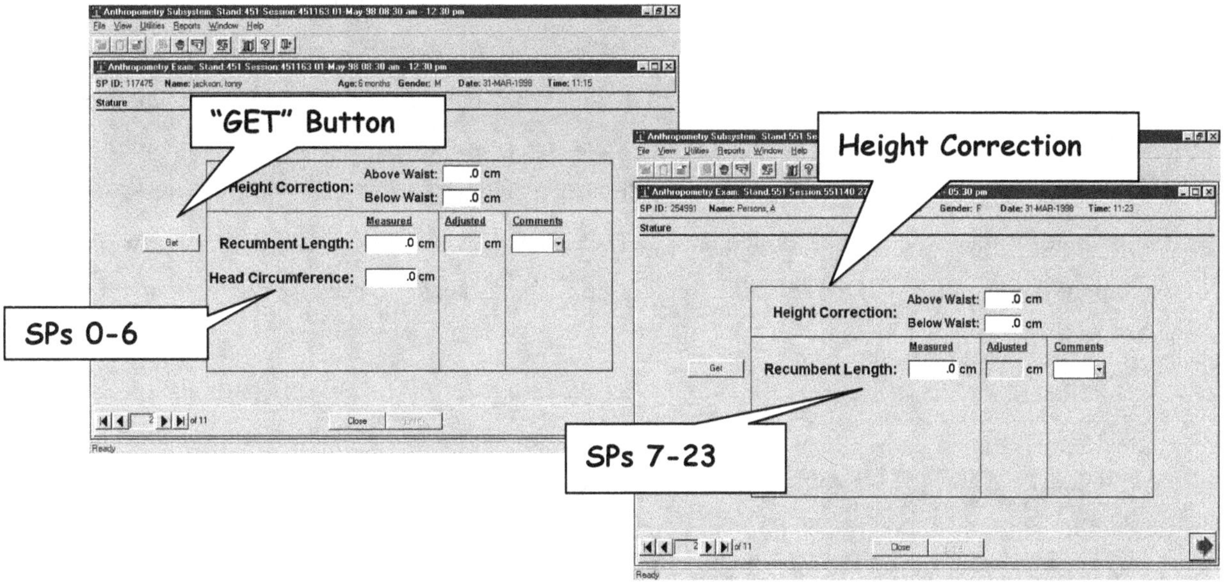

There are two fields for Height Correction located at the top of the screen. If an SP is wearing a hairpiece such as a barrette, braids, or a bun that they decline to remove for the measure, the examiner will measure the hairpiece with a ruler and you will enter the measure in the *Height Correction: Above Waist* field. Likewise, if an SP declines to remove his or her shoes when being measured, the examiner will measure the height of the heels and you will enter it into the *Height Correction: Below Waist* field.

You will capture the recumbent length and the standing height automatically when you click on the "Get" button to the left of the measure. After each measure is captured or entered into the system, a voice will be activated that says the measurement aloud for confirmation.

There are three columns on the screen: Measured, Adjusted, and Comments. The system will display the captured height in the Measured column. The system will then automatically calculate the adjusted values. Both *Height Correction: Above Waist* and *Height Correction: Below Waist* will be subtracted from the Standing Height measured value. The adjusted height will be displayed in the Adjusted column. If comments are needed for any measure, you will click on the down arrow to the right of the corresponding Comments box and a drop-down list will appear. If you could not obtain a height you must enter either CNO (could not obtain), HTO (hard to obtain), or EC (exceeds capacity). If a measurement was captured but the examiner did not think it was accurate because the SP was not straight, enter NS (not straight).

Exhibit 3-20. Stature screens, 3 columns

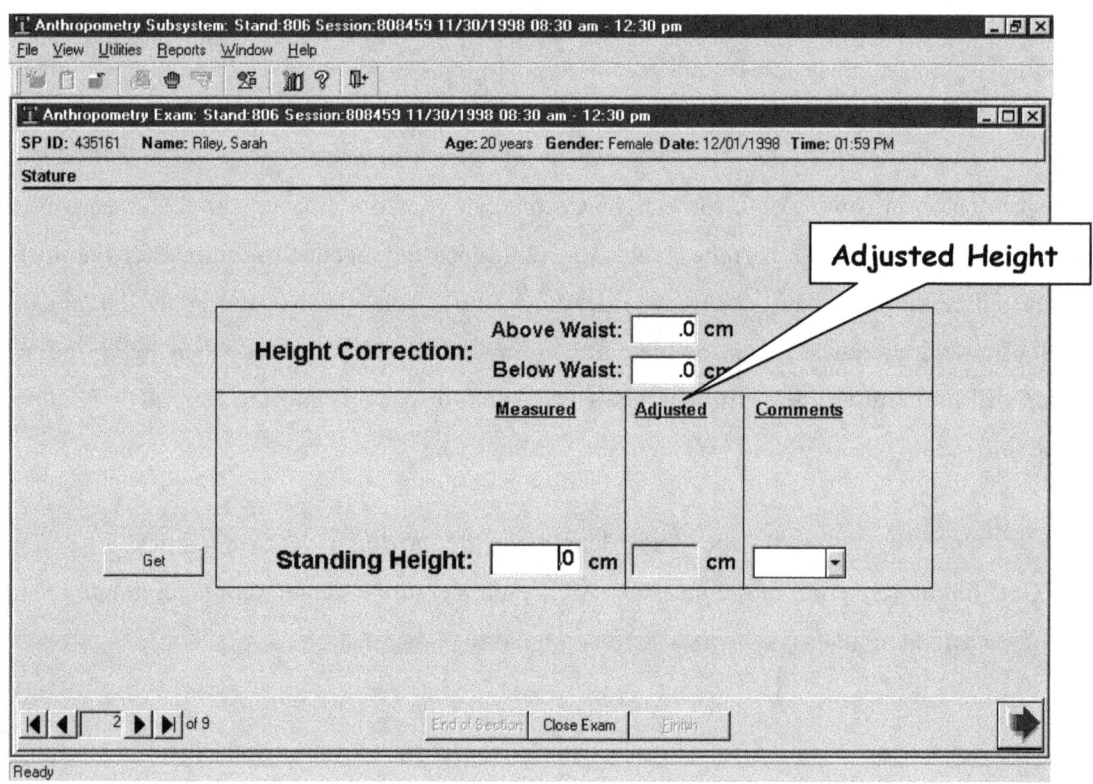

### 3.3.2.4 Sitting Measures Screen

The next screen is **Sitting Measures**. This screen will be displayed for all SPs 8 years of age or older. This screen displays two measures: Upper Leg Length and Max-Calf Circumference. After you enter the first measurement in the screen, press the **Tab** button on the keyboard to move the cursor to the next measurement field. The system will repeat aloud each measurement as it is entered.

After you have entered the Upper Leg Length, the system will calculate the midpoint of the upper leg length and say it aloud. You (the recorder) will then mark the Upper leg midpoint with a cosmetic pencil for the examiner.

Exhibit 3-21. Sitting Measures screens

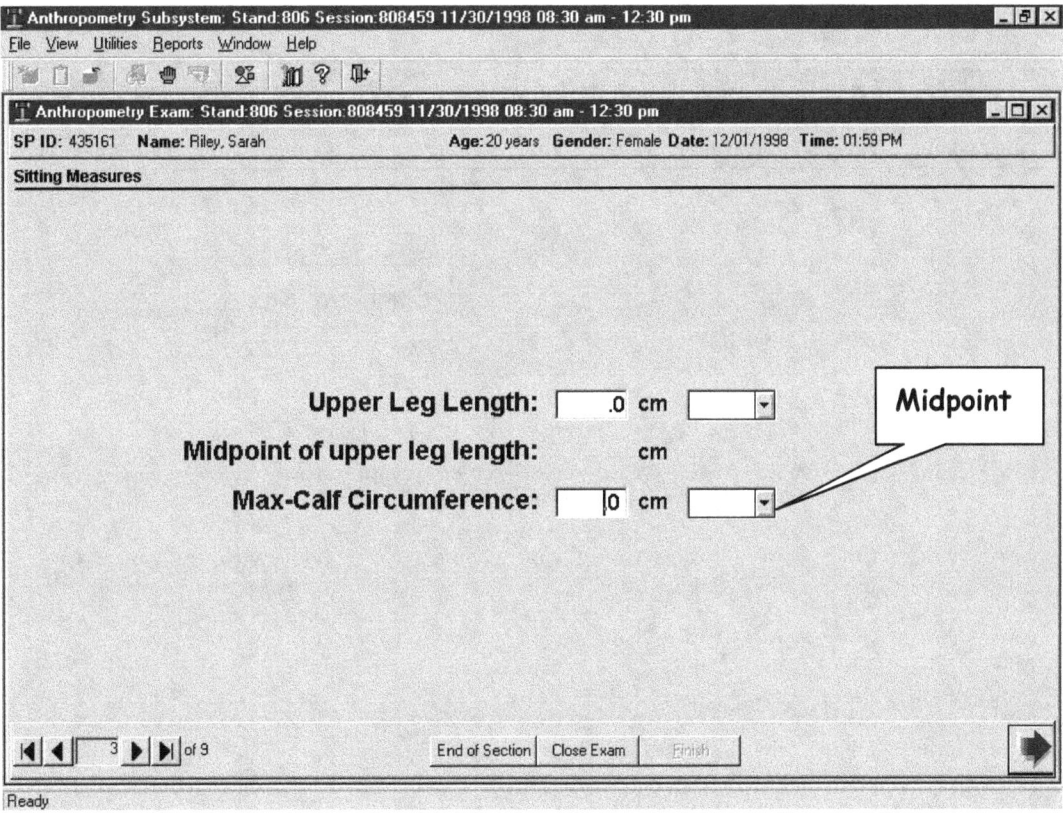

### 3.3.2.5 Upper Arm Length Screen

The next screen is **Upper Arm Length**. This screen will be displayed for all SPs aged 2 months or older. After you enter the measure in the field, the system will first repeat the measure aloud, and then calculate and say aloud the midpoint of the upper arm length. You (the recorder) will then mark the Upper arm midpoint with a cosmetic pencil for the examiner.

If you cannot obtain the measure for some reason (e.g., respondent refuses the measure), you must enter the comment "CNO" for "Could not obtain" in the Comment box.

Exhibit 3-22. Upper Arm Length screen

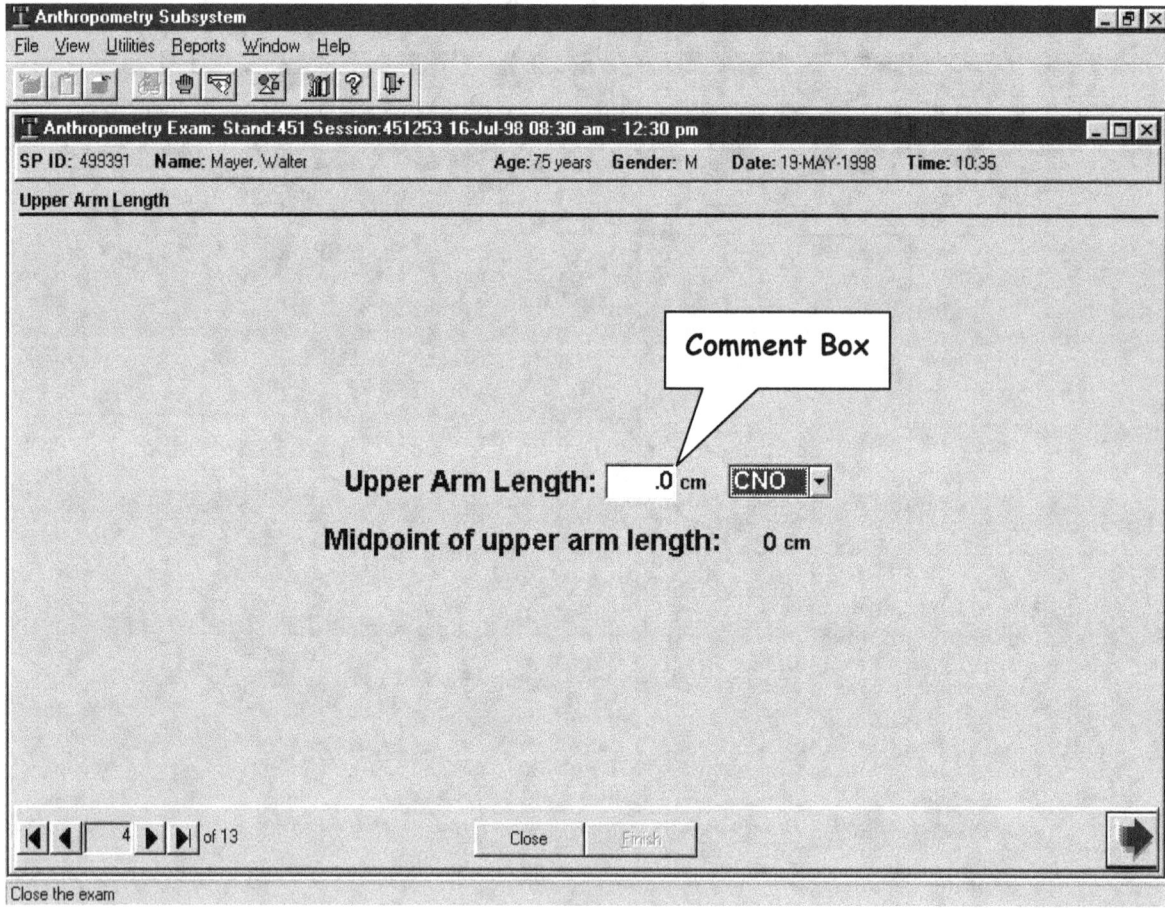

**3.3.2.6    Circumference Measures Screen**

The **Circumference Measures** screen will be displayed for all SPs 2 months or older. This screen contains four measures: Maximal Calf Circumference, Arm Circumference, Waist Circumference, and Thigh Circumference. Only the arm circumference field is activated for SPs 2-23 months old. The system will repeat aloud each measure after it is entered. Use the **Tab** button on the keyboard to move the cursor to the next measurement box.

Exhibit 3-23. Circumference Measures screens

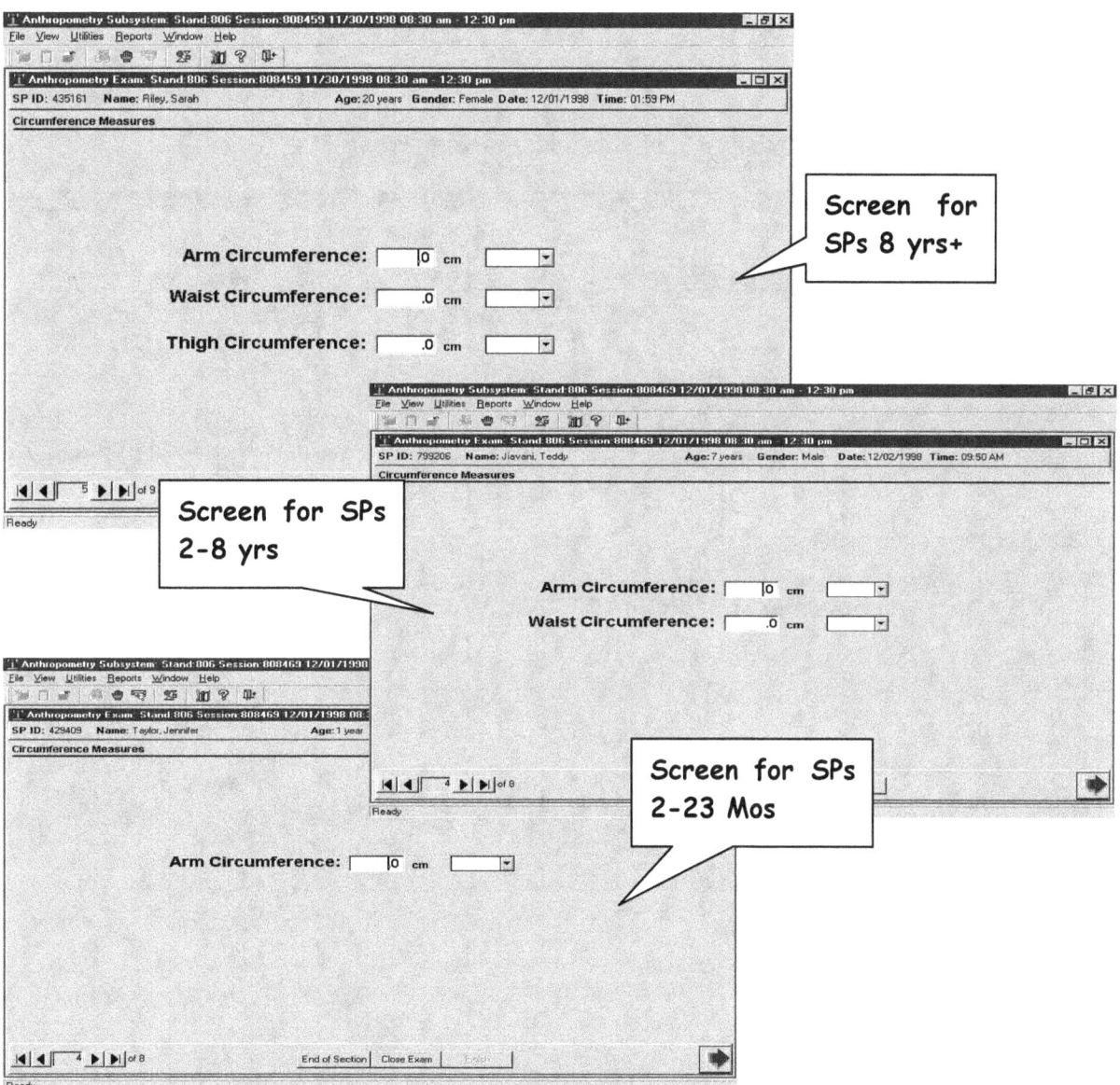

### 3.3.2.7 Skinfold Measures Screen

The **Skinfold Measures** screen will be displayed for all SPs 2 months and older. Two skinfold measurements will be collected on this screen: Triceps skinfold and Subscapular skinfold. After entering each measurement, the system will repeat aloud the measure for confirmation. Use the Tab button on the keyboard to move the cursor to the next measurement box. Notice that you can enter a comment for any or all of the skinfold measures. The upper limit of the calipers is 45 mm; the system will not allow any measurements greater than 45 mm to be entered. If you cannot obtain a measure, either because the SP refused the measure or the skinfold was too large for the caliper, you must enter a comment before leaving the screen.

Exhibit 3-24. Skinfold Measures screens

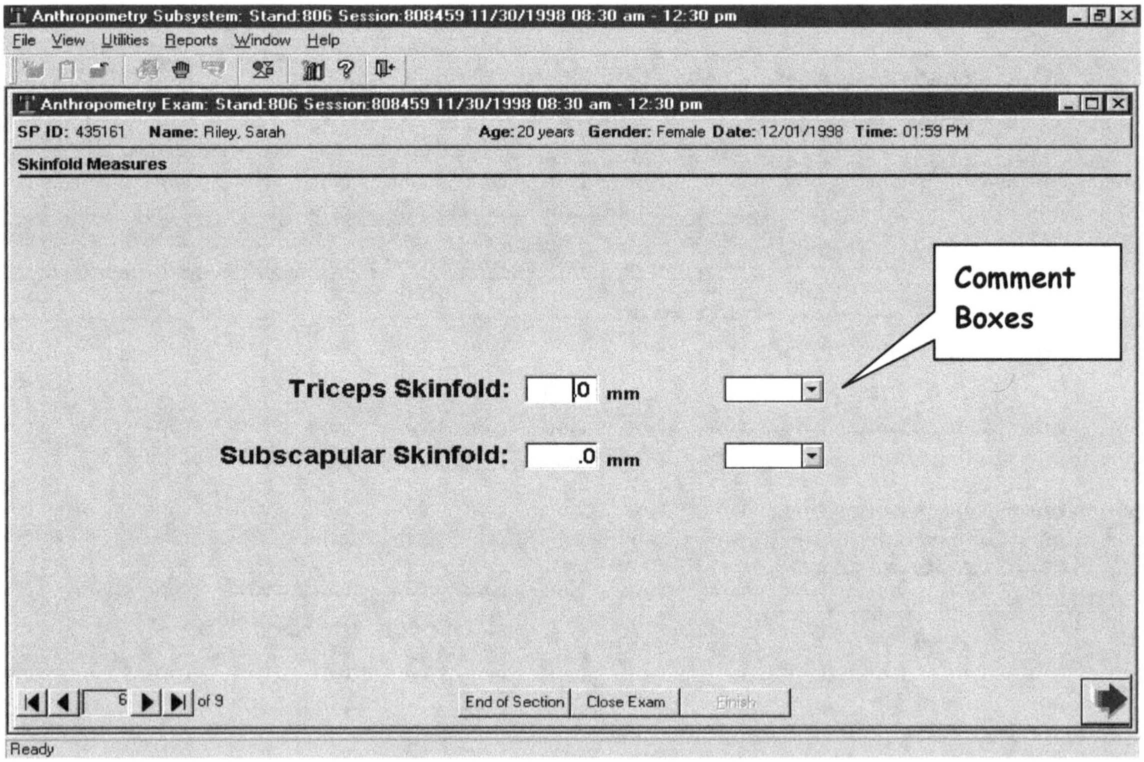

### 3.3.2.8    SP Information Screen

The next screen is **SP Information**. This screen displays the question "Do you want to know your height and weight?" Read the question to the SP and click on either "Yes" or "No." If you select "Yes," two pop-up boxes will appear. These boxes display the SP's weight and height, including the metric equivalents of each measurement. If you select "No," the system moves to the Amputations screen.

Exhibit 3-25. SP Information screen

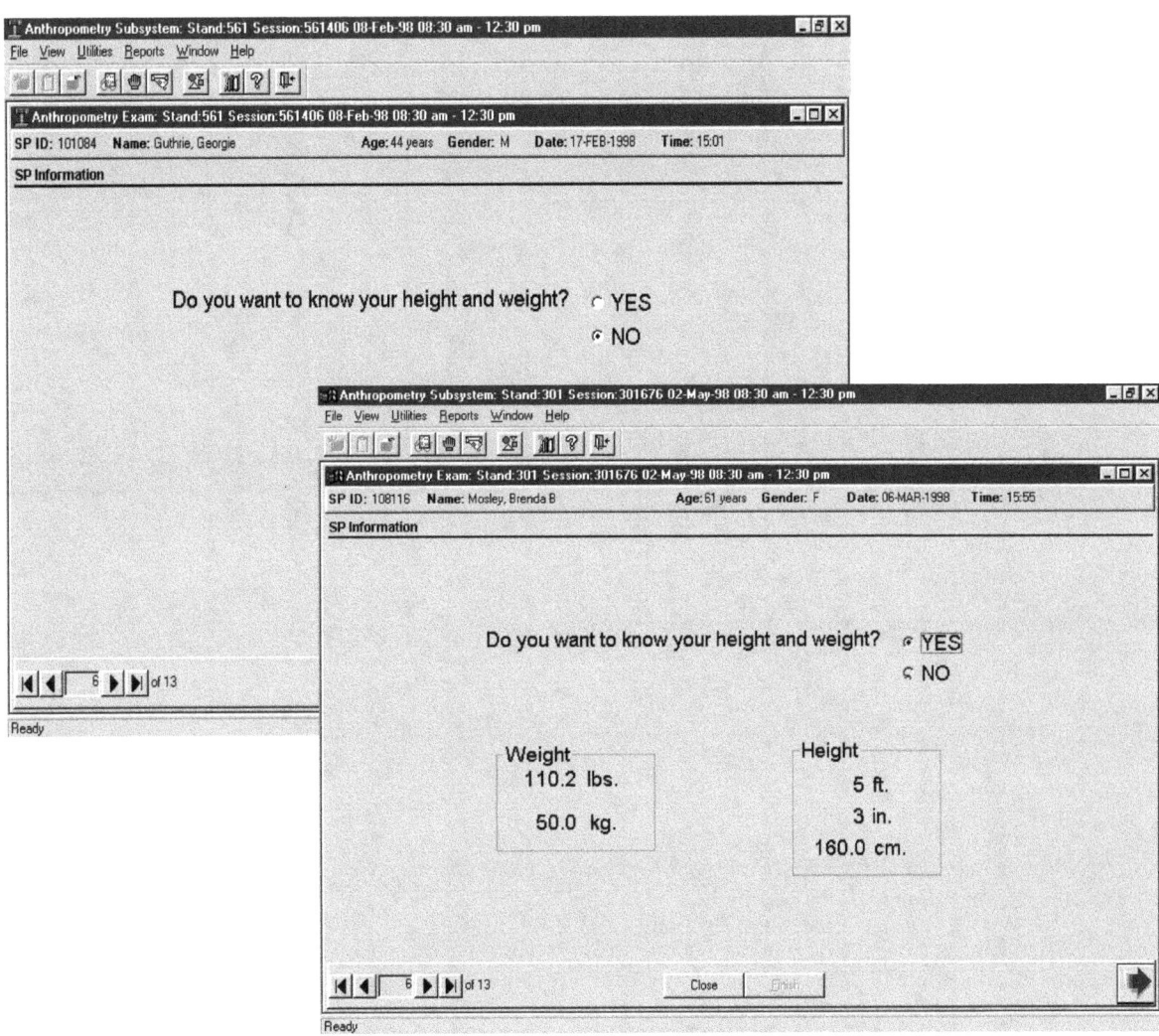

### 3.3.2.9 Amputations Screen

The next screen is **Amputations**. "Yes" and "No" options are displayed and you will choose accordingly. If you click on "Yes," the system automatically will add four questions to the screen: Upper Right Extremity?, Upper Left Extremity?, Lower Right Extremity?, and Lower Left Extremity? You must choose from one of the three options that follow for each question: "Yes," "No," and "Could not obtain." If you click on "Yes" for either of the upper extremities, the system will automatically add two questions to the screen: Above Elbow? and Below Elbow?; if you click "Yes" for either of the lower extremities, the system will automatically add the options Above Knee? and Below Knee? to the screen. You must choose one of these options each time you click "Yes" for an extremity.

Exhibit 3-26. Amputations screens

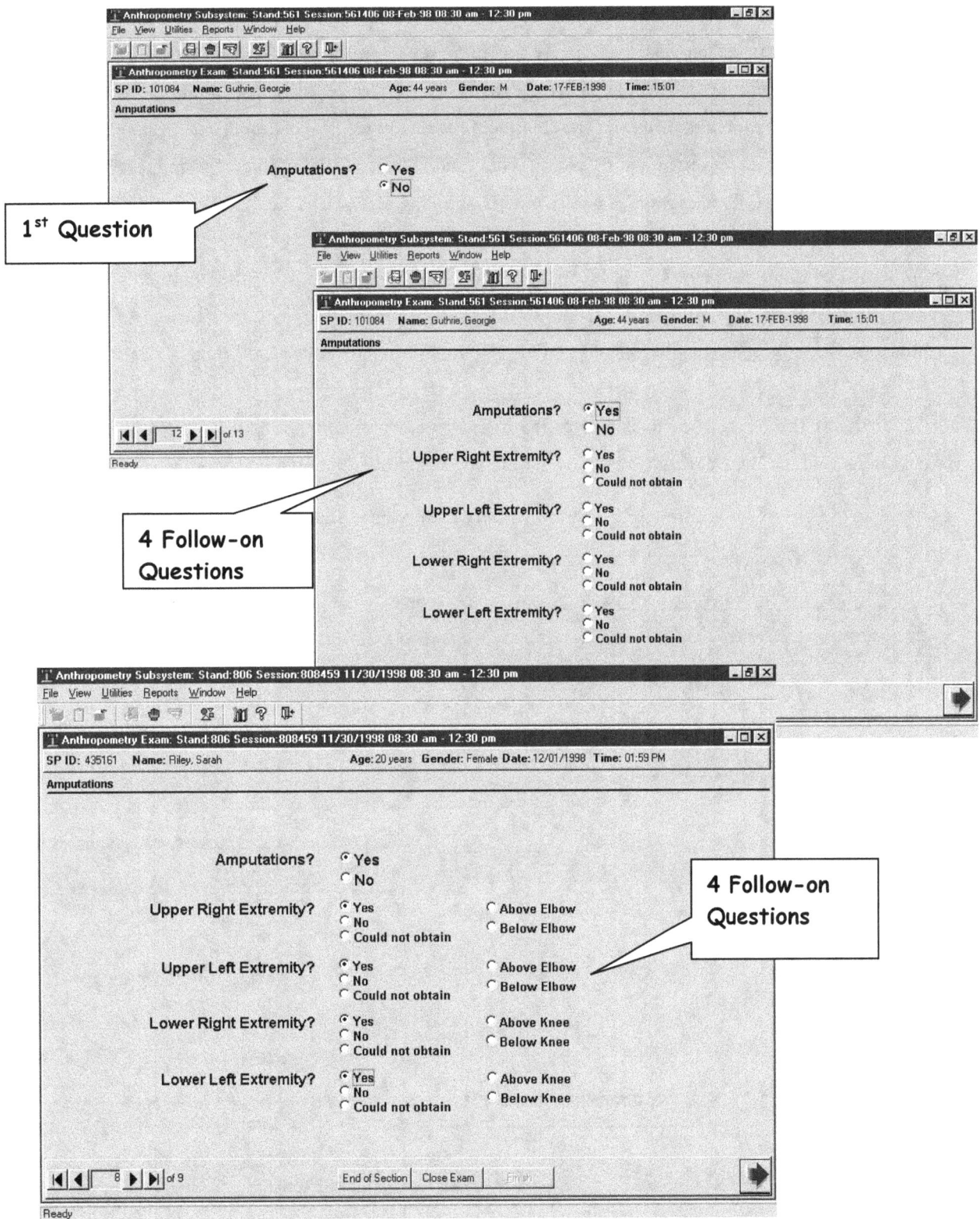

### 3.3.2.10 Anthropometry Component Status Screen

The last screen displayed is **Anthropometry Component Status**. This screen has three options: Complete, Partial, and Not Done. If the status is Partial or Not Done, you must enter a comment. Click on the down arrow to the right of the Comments box to make a selection. There are eight comments to choose from: safety exclusion, SP refusal, no time, physical limitation, communication problem, equipment failure, SP ill/emergency, or interrupted. You may also select the "Other, specify" comment. If you choose the "Other, specify" comment you must enter text into the "Other text" field to describe the comment. The eight comments in the Comments box should cover most of the comments you need to make. Only use the "Other, specify" comment if your comment does not fit into one of the defined comments. Be as brief as possible when you type a comment in the "Other text" field.

If the SP refuses to complete the anthropometry examination in its entirety, an abridged examination will be done during which only stature and weight will be obtained.

Exhibit 3-27. Anthropometry Component Status screen

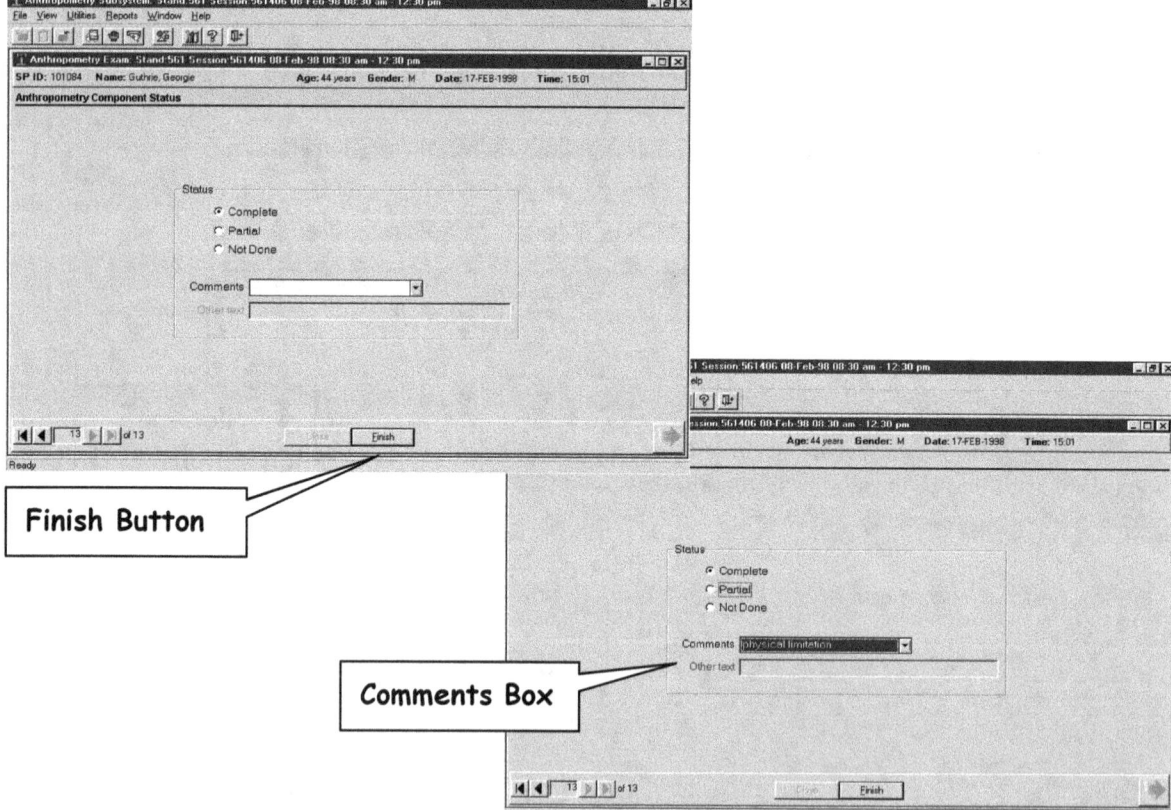

## 3.4    Postexamination Procedures

After completion of the body measurement examination, the examiner should remove all cosmetic pencil marks from the SP's skin with alcohol or baby oil on a piece of gauze. Then, if ISIS determines that the SP is PAM-eligible, the Finish box on the Anthropometry Component Status Screen will be disabled and the examiner will click the large arrow to advance the screen, initiating PAM. However, if ISIS determines that the SP is ineligible for the PAM component, the examiner will simply click the Finish box to end the examination. One of the technologists should direct or accompany the SP to his or her next examination as per MEC procedures.

# 4. QUALITY CONTROL

Quality control procedures for body measurements are extremely important and must be observed. The most common errors in anthropometrics are body positioning, reading measurements, and recording. In order to minimize these errors, standard procedures for obtaining measurements are described in this manual. The goal of the training session is to standardize all examiners to these procedures. Errors made in measuring technique are also minimized by the recorder's role in assisting the examiner. The recorder assists the examiner with positioning of the SP and the examiner's reading process. Reading errors frequently occur as a result of parallax, the phenomenon where an observer sees a different value on a measuring device depending on the angle from which it is viewed. Again, standardization in training will help alleviate this problem.

## 4.1    Examination Screens

The examination screens are designed to be as recorder-friendly as possible and at the same time ensure that the data entered are as accurate as possible. Following are some quality-control features of the ISIS system:

- The weight, length, and height measurements are directly entered into the computer system by clicking on the "Get" buttons.

- You must enter a number or a comment in every field before the program will let you move to the next screen.

- When you move to a new screen, the cursor will be in the correct field for data entry.

- A computer voice repeats each measure after it is entered to verify the measure.

## 4.2    Automated System

The automated system is designed to function as a quality control measure by minimizing possible measuring and recording errors. Edit ranges have been set for all measurements. If a measurement does not fall within the 1st and 99th percentile based on NHANES III data, the system will display an "out of range" message prompting the examiner to recheck the measurement to ensure that it is the "correct" value. It is possible that some SPs (i.e., very small or very large) will not be within the "normal" ranges. Therefore, the examiner and recorder must verify the original measurement value.

It is extremely important to measure skinfolds accurately. Even after extensive practice it is possible to make errors due to slight misplacement of the caliper or misreading the dial. Therefore it is important that examiners are well versed in the examination protocol and take care in obtaining each measurement precisely.

The system also ensures that the placement of decimal points and the number of digits entered are correct. For instance, if the number of positions entered for a measurement exceeds the number of positions allowed for a measurement, it cannot be entered.

## 4.3     Procedures for Using Hard Copy Forms to Enter Measurements

If the automated system fails during a session, contact the data manager. If the data manager is unable to correct the problem, perform the examination as usual and enter the measurements on the Body Measures Recording Form (see Appendix A). Several copies of this form should be kept in a drawer in the room; blank forms can be accessed by the data manager in the blank forms directory. Use extra care when entering measures on hard copy to minimize the possibility of errors. The MEC manager should notify the home office of the situation as quickly as possible. The home office will take steps to correct the problem with the automated system and give directions to fax the hard copy forms so the data can be entered into the system.

## 4.4     Equipment Calibrations

Routine calibrations and checks of the body measurement equipment ensure that the equipment is standardized and producing accurate measures.

## 4.5    Review, Observations, and Replication

Technologists will be periodically observed by the body measurement consultant to ensure standardization. The consultant will review with the technologists any deviations from the protocol.

**Replication.** Different types of replicates will be utilized in the current NHANES as quality control measures:

- **Complete Replicates** - Replicates who will be scheduled from the pool of volunteers for a complete reexamination at the MEC.

- **"Expert" Replicates** - These are the replications performed by experts, i.e., the body measurement consultant.

## 4.6    Refresher Sessions

Refresher or retraining sessions will be scheduled when major changes in protocol are introduced or when a lack of standardization is observed among the technologists.

# 5. SAFETY PROCEDURES

## 5.1    Equipment Precautions

All equipment in the body measurement room should be checked, maintained, and cleaned on a regular basis to protect the equipment, the SP, and the technologist. If any equipment is broken or starts to break, discontinue using it and notify the MEC manager. Broken equipment should be removed from the body measurement room and/or central areas in the MEC.

## 5.2    SP Movement and Positioning

The process of taking body measurements does not impose any physical harm or risk to the SP. However, there are certain precautions to be observed by the technologists due to specific positioning for the varied measurement components.

SPs that seem unsteady on their feet should be encouraged to hold onto the diagonal bar while their weight is taken, and the horizontal bar while the circumferences and skinfold measurements are taken.

Performing body measurements on children requires additional safety precautions and monitoring. Children in the body measurement room require constant supervision by the technologists. All anthropometric equipment should be placed out of reach of the smaller children. When using the recumbent length board or the body measurement table, children must be carefully held by the technologist to prevent any falls. Keep in mind that babies and small children tend to flip themselves over very quickly. Place equipment baskets low enough on the wall to prevent the possibility of items falling onto an infant on the recumbent length board. NEVER leave an infant/child unattended on the recumbent length board. Again, it is the technologist's responsibility to carefully explain and monitor the body measurement procedures to adequately protect the SPs from any physical injury.

## 5.3        Emergency Procedures

Procedures for medical emergencies and other types of emergency situations are discussed in the Standardized Procedures.

# 6. PHYSICAL ACTIVITY MONITOR

## 6.1        Introduction

The purpose of the Physical Activity Monitor component (PAMC) is to assess the physical activity levels of NHANES examinees 6+ years of age. Approximately 4,000 individuals are expected to participate in this component annually. NHANES examinees wear a physical activity monitor (PAM) to examine physical activity patterns over a 7-day monitoring period. The monitors detect locomotion-type activities such as walking or jogging. The monitors provide a means of capturing nonstructured activities that are often difficult for survey respondents (SPs) to self-report. Minors are included in this study because they are an important target population group for the NHANES nutrition assessment component. Physical activity data are linked to other household interview and health component data and are used to track changes that occur in body weight, and functional, bone, and health statuses over time.

From a public health perspective, there is compelling data to show that physical inactivity is an independent risk factor for coronary heart disease (Berlin and Colditz, 1990). In the United States, a significant percentage of deaths from coronary heart disease, colon cancer, and Type 2 diabetes are attributable to sedentary lifestyle (Blair and Morrow, Jr., 1998). Even moderate-intensity activity is beneficial to overall health (Pate, JAMA, 1995) because it contributes to improved glucose tolerance and blood lipid profile levels. Additionally, NHANES 1999-2000 data demonstrates continued increases in the prevalence of obesity and overweight among all age groups of Americans.

The American College of Sports Medicine, the Centers for Disease Control and Prevention, the American Heart Association, the National Institutes of Health, and the President's Council on Physical Fitness and Sports recommend regular, moderate-intensity physical activity. *The U.S. Surgeon General's Report on Physical Activity and Health* reported that more than 60 percent of Americans do not engage in regular physical activity and that 25 percent do not engage in any activity (DHHS, 1996). The report reaffirmed the importance of regular moderate or vigorous-intensity activity. Until now, it has been difficult to assess actual physical activity levels in free-living populations because the cost and complexity of performing the monitoring tasks required to obtain this information were prohibitive. Furthermore, physical activity data on children, particularly children in the 6-11 year age group are lacking. Proxy information on physical activity levels among youth are not useful because children spend large amounts of time away from home and they engage in sporadic periods of activity that are difficult to document, let alone quantify. Reliable, accurate methods are now available to assess physical activity levels in large groups of free-living individuals.

NHANES uses the CSA/MTI accelerometer model 7164 to monitor physical activity. The CSA/MTI monitor has a long record of accomplishment in clinical and community-based physical activity studies. The monitor enables researchers to examine the duration of physical activity at varying levels of intensity. In addition, the monitors have a step counter feature that provides another objective measure of physical activity. For example, some countries have set physical activity recommendations for population groups that are based upon a certain number of steps traveled per day.

### 6.1.1    Overview of the Health Technologist's Responsibilities

The PAM component is the second section in the body measures examination. The appropriate PAM screens display after the body measures section screen.

MEC health technologists recruit SPs aged 6+ to wear the physical activity monitor for 7 days. They instruct the SP to wear the PAM under or against light clothing on the right hip, during waking hours for seven (7) full days, beginning the day after their MEC examination. The health technologist initializes the monitor using the reader interface unit (RIU), places it on a removable elastic belt that has a Velcro closure and fits the belt on the SP. The monitors are water resistant, but not waterproof and should be removed before swimming, showering, or bathing. The health technologist provides verbal and written instructions to the SP to reinforce these precautions.

The health technologist affixes a self-sticking label on the PAM. This label includes the participant's name to minimize confusion when multiple study participants reside in the same household. The NHANES logo and a toll-free "800" telephone number is embossed on the monitor case. Assistance will be provided by telephone if questions or problems arise during the study. English and Spanish speaking staff members are available to answer questions that arise during the study.

## 6.1.2    Overview of the Home Office Responsibilities

Upon completion of the 7-day test period, survey participants mail the PAM device to the NHANES warehouse using a postage-paid padded envelope. Separate return mailing envelopes are provided for each survey participant's PAM device. Once the monitor is received at the home office, the warehouse staff downloads the data and cleans and calibrates each monitor. The warehouse staff checks the battery life and installs new batteries, when indicated. Monitors are recycled.

Participants receive a reminder postcard at the end of the data collection period (7-8 days after the MEC exam). Upon receipt of the monitor back at the home office, a remuneration check for forty ($40) dollars is mailed to the participant.

If the monitor is not returned within 12 days post-MEC exam, reminder contacts are initiated by the Westat phone center offices in Gaithersburg, MD. Monitors not returned within 12 days after the MEC exam constitute a broken appointment. If a monitor is overdue, then a reminder notice displays at the end of the Dietary Phone Followup (DPFU) Interview. The dietary interviewer reminds the SP that they should return the monitor.

## 6.2     Equipment and Supplies

The body measurements room contains the PAM reader interface unit and the Intermec thermal transfer printer. At the start and end of each stand, take a complete inventory using the established inventory procedures.

The equipment and supplies used in the PAMC are listed in Exhibit 6-1.

Exhibit 6-1. Equipment and supplies – physical activity monitor

| MEC | |
|---|---|
| PAMC kits | Reader interface unit |
|    Physical activity monitor | Lister scissors |
|    Elastic belt with Velcro® closure (80 inches) | Placebo monitor for demonstration |
|    Information sheet | Intermec thermal transfer printer |
|    2 Informational flyers from NCHS | Intermec labels |
|    Padded mailers | Intermec thermal transfer ribbon |

| Warehouse | |
|---|---|
|    Screwdriver | Reader interface unit |
|    Duracell batteries | Calibrator |

### 6.2.1    Actigraph Monitors

The activity monitor (Actigraph) is a single axis accelerometer that has been programmed to detect normal human motion and reject motion from other sources (see picture below). The data collected by the monitor is a series of numbers representing a level or intensity of activity in a set period of time (1-minute intervals). The accelerometer sensor element is not located in the center of the case but it is located at the end of the case opposite the end of the notch. For this reason, consistent orientation of the monitor on the belt and the belt on the SP is critical. The monitor runs on a CR2430 coin-cell lithium battery.

Actigraph Activity Monitor — Notch

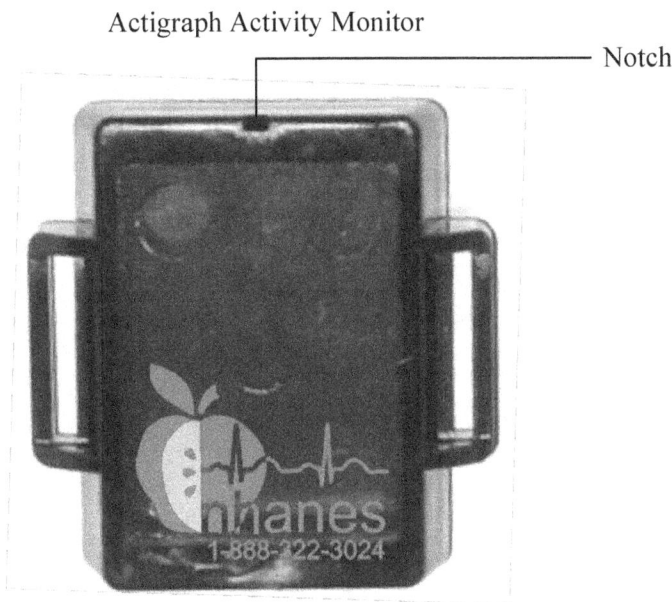

### 6.2.2    Reader Interface Unit

The activity monitor interfaces with a computer using a reader interface unit (RIU) connected to the computer in the phlebotomy room. The activity monitor must be placed correctly on the RIU in order for the monitor to be initialized. The activity monitor should be placed with the back cover and screws facing up. The notched end of the activity monitor should be directly over the finger access slot in the front wall of the RIU.

### 6.2.3     Warehouse Responsibilities

The warehouse staff assembles PAMC kits. Each PAMC kit consists of one activity monitor, one elastic belt, one information sheet, and two copies of an informational flyer in a padded return envelope. The padded envelope is labeled with a business reply postage-paid label.

### 6.3     Overview

The coordinator tracks each SP through the MEC using the coordinator system. This system tracks the SP throughout the exam, including arrival, location during the session, and exit. The coordinator uses this system to direct the SP to the appropriate workstations in the MEC and to determine if all the appropriate examinations are complete. The MEC coordinator monitors exam component status using responses from examination stations.

The NHANES dietary interview proxy rules apply to the PAM component for wearing and removing the monitors during the study. Proxies (preferably a parent or guardian) assist survey participants who are 6-11 years of age at the time of the examination. Respondents 12 years of age and older receive instructions on how to wear their monitor and remove the monitor before going to bed.

Each SP receives a bar-coded ID bracelet upon arrival at the MEC. The bracelet remains on the SP throughout the session. This bracelet contains the SP's ID number in bar code and eye-readable format. The health technologist "wands" the bracelet bar code with a bar code scanner (wand) to log the SP into the phlebotomy component. If necessary, the ID number can be entered manually by reading it from the bracelet.

The health technologists are responsible for completing sections within the body measures exam:

- Body measures; and
- Physical activity monitor.

Access the body measures application and open the body measures exam. Log the SP into phlebotomy by scanning the bar code on the SP ID bracelet or manually typing the SP ID when the SP arrives in the examination room.

Complete the body measures examination procedure and then recruit SPs aged 6+ to wear the physical activity monitor for 7 days. Explain the purpose of this component and how to wear and return the monitor. Instruct the SP to wear the PAM under or against light clothing on the right hip, during waking hours for seven (7) full days, beginning the day after their MEC examination. Initialize the monitor, place it on a removable elastic belt that has a Velcro closure, and fit the belt on the SP. The monitors are water resistant, but not waterproof and should be removed before swimming, showering, or bathing. Provide verbal and written instructions to the SP to reinforce these precautions.

### 6.3.1    PAMC Kits

Each SP will receive a Velcro® stretch belt onto which the monitor is attached. The belts come in one size – 80 inches. The health technologist cuts the belt to the approximate size, places the monitor on the belt, fits the belt on the SP, and trims the belt.

Each SP will be given:

- One monitor on a Velcro® elastic belt;

- Two copies of an informational flyer on survey letterhead explaining the activity monitor;

- One copy of an information sheet that summarizes the details relating to the monitor; and

- One padded envelope (with the postage-paid sticker) to use when returning the monitor.

### 6.4    Gaining Cooperation

The coordinator introduces the SP to the examination and briefly explains the examination process. The coordinator can answer any general questions the SP has about the phlebotomy exam, including the PAMC. However, the health technologists must be prepared to answer all the questions the SP poses about the PAM procedure. In addition, the health technologist must convince the SP of the importance of cooperating in the PAM component. (SPs do not receive any results.)

If an SP initially refuses the component, then ask questions to determine the reason for the refusal and try to address any concerns the SP has in order to have him or her complete the component. Provide reassurance and encouragement. If he or she still refuses, code the exam as an SP refusal. If the SP is planning to be out of the country for the next few weeks, assess his or her ability to remember to return the monitor. To address SP's concerns effectively, know the following information about the procedures used for the study:

**Safety**

- There is no reason to exclude mentally impaired or handicapped individuals who are mobile. A proxy respondent can assist mentally challenged individuals with their monitors. Exclude individuals who use a wheelchair.

- There are no known risks associated with use of the monitors. The activity monitor is not waterproof but if the monitor accidentally gets wet, this does not pose a danger. The Actigraph is powered by a 3-volt watch battery, which does not present a shock hazard when worn in a wet environment. The battery is housed securely inside the device and a special screwdriver is required to open the device. The PAM device does not emit radiation, electrical current, vibration, or heat and it can be worn under clothing without causing discomfort or embarrassment.

  **Note to MEC staff:** Do not attempt to open the monitor. The screws are tiny and delicate. The home office staff has special equipment to use when opening the cases.

- There is a small risk of accidental choking if the device is removed from the web belt and left within reach of small children or pets. The CSA/MTI device dimensions are 2 inches x 1.5 inches x ½ inch. The device is intended to be worn or stored securely fastened to a long, ¾ -inch wide belt at all times. There is no reason for the device to be removed from the belt.

- The other potential hazard is that the waist belt could catch on something. The belt should be securely fastened to the waist-hip area. Information about potential safety concerns will be included in written materials that are given to the survey participants and proxies and included in the scripts that are used by staff in the MEC.

- The PAM will not interfere with a pacemaker.

## 6.4.1      Answering Questions

**1.      Will the monitor harm me in any way?**

No, the monitor will not harm you in any way. A small watch battery that is securely housed in the device powers the monitor. The monitor does not emit radiation, electrical current, vibration, or heat and it can be worn under your clothing without causing discomfort or embarrassment.

**2.      I play a team sport and we are not allowed to wear jewelry. How do I explain this to my coach?**

We are providing you with two copies of an informational flyer to show anyone who asks about your participation in this study. Keep the letter with you, so you can respond to questions.

**3.      What do I need to do if I have to go through a metal detector (at airport, school, government building)?**

Please take the belt off and put it in the bin to be screened. This will not harm the monitor in any way. In addition, please keep the informational flyer we provided to show security personnel.

**4.      I swim a lot, what do I need to do?**

Do not wear the monitor while swimming. The monitors should not get wet.

**5.      What do I do if I lose the envelope?**

Call the toll-free number we provided you and another mailer envelope will be sent to your home.

**6.      I will be out-of-town during the next week.**

It is OK to participate while you are out-of-town. You can mail the monitor back to us from any location within the United States.

## 6.4.2      Background

It is helpful to understand the NCI research activities in the area of physical activity. Use this information to answer questions.

The Division of Cancer Control and Population Sciences conducts a variety of epidemiological, surveillance, and behavioral research activities to explore the association between physical activity and a number of cancer sites. The Division's research objectives are posted on their web site: http://dccps.nci.nih.gov/DECC/dwpa_pa.html. The areas of research that are especially relevant to NHANES include:

- The characteristics of physical activity such as frequency, intensity, and types of activities people engage in—topics that are included in NHANES questionnaires are of interest;

- Methodological research interests include development of improved, standardized methods for assessment of physical activity, especially those for lifetime history, adolescent, and young adult physical activity; and

- The association of physical activity with site-specific cancer for diverse populations defined by age, income, education, and race or ethnicity.

In the area of surveillance, and as noted in the *Surgeon General's Report on Physical Activity and Health* (1996):

- Develop methods to monitor patterns of regular, moderate physical activity; and

- Improve the validity and comparability of self-reported physical activity in national surveys.

Behavioral research targets the following:

- Examine the impact of physical activity and physical activity interventions on other cancer-related risk behaviors; and

- Examine the impact of psychosocial sequelae of survivorship on weight, weight management, physical activity, and diet.

## 6.5 Exclusions

There are only a few reasons to exclude an SP from this component. They are:

- The SP's girth is too large to accommodate the belt. This includes pregnant SPs when the belt will not fit around their waist. Pregnancy alone is not an exclusion. SPs are excluded only if their waists are too big for the belt;

- The SP is in a wheelchair; and

- The SP had recent abdominal surgery.

## 6.6 Recruiting SPs Who Do Not Speak English

When the health technologist attempts to recruit an SP who does not speak English and the health technologist does not speak the language of the SP, a translator who does speak the language of the SP assists the health technologist.

The translator stays with the health technologist and the SP **for the entire procedure**. It is very important that the health technologist be able to communicate with the SP if the SP becomes ill during the procedure.

## 6.7 Recruit the SP

The Physical Activity Monitor slide displays after the Body Measures section status slide.

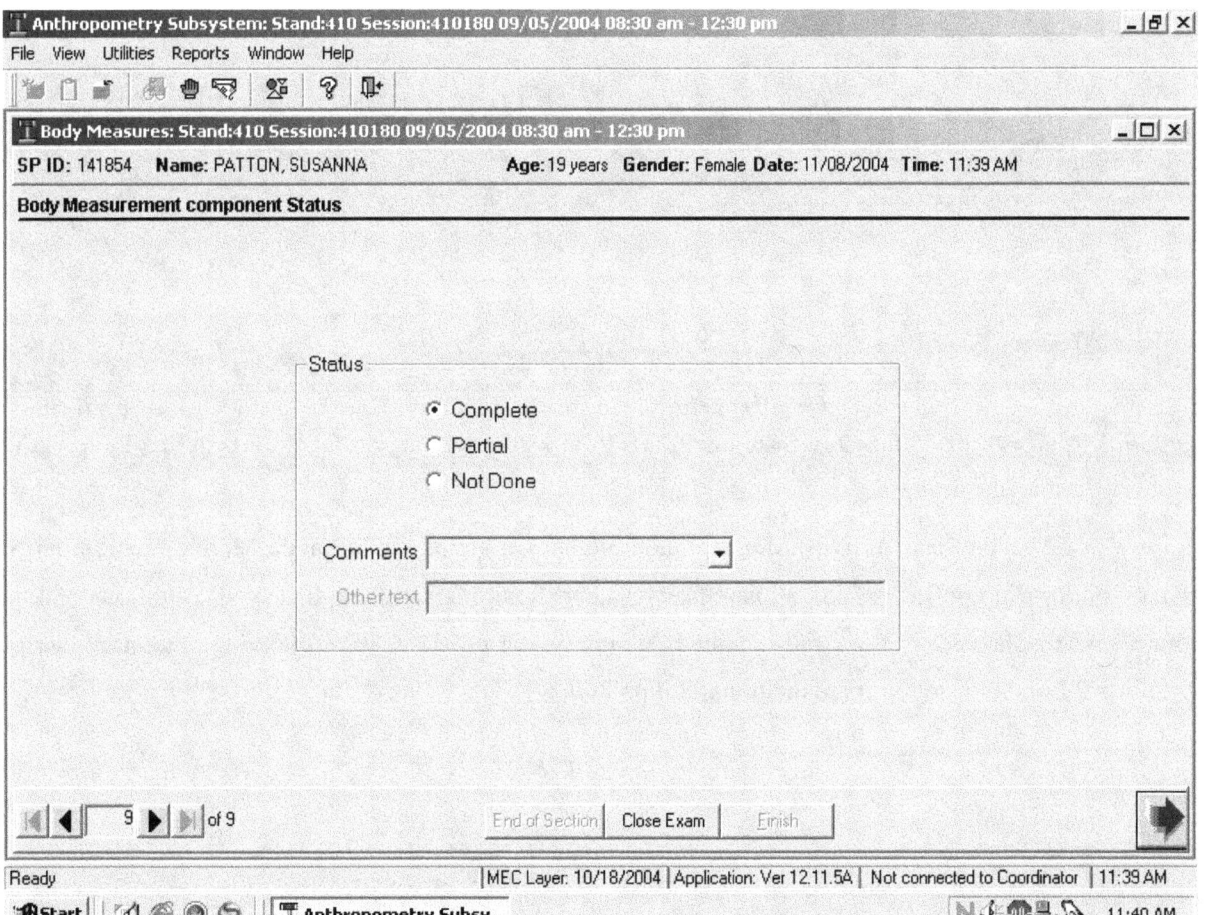

Introduce the PAM as the "next component" in the body measures exam. Simply state that the SP has been selected for this component.

The Physical Activity Monitor slide displays after the body measures section status slide.

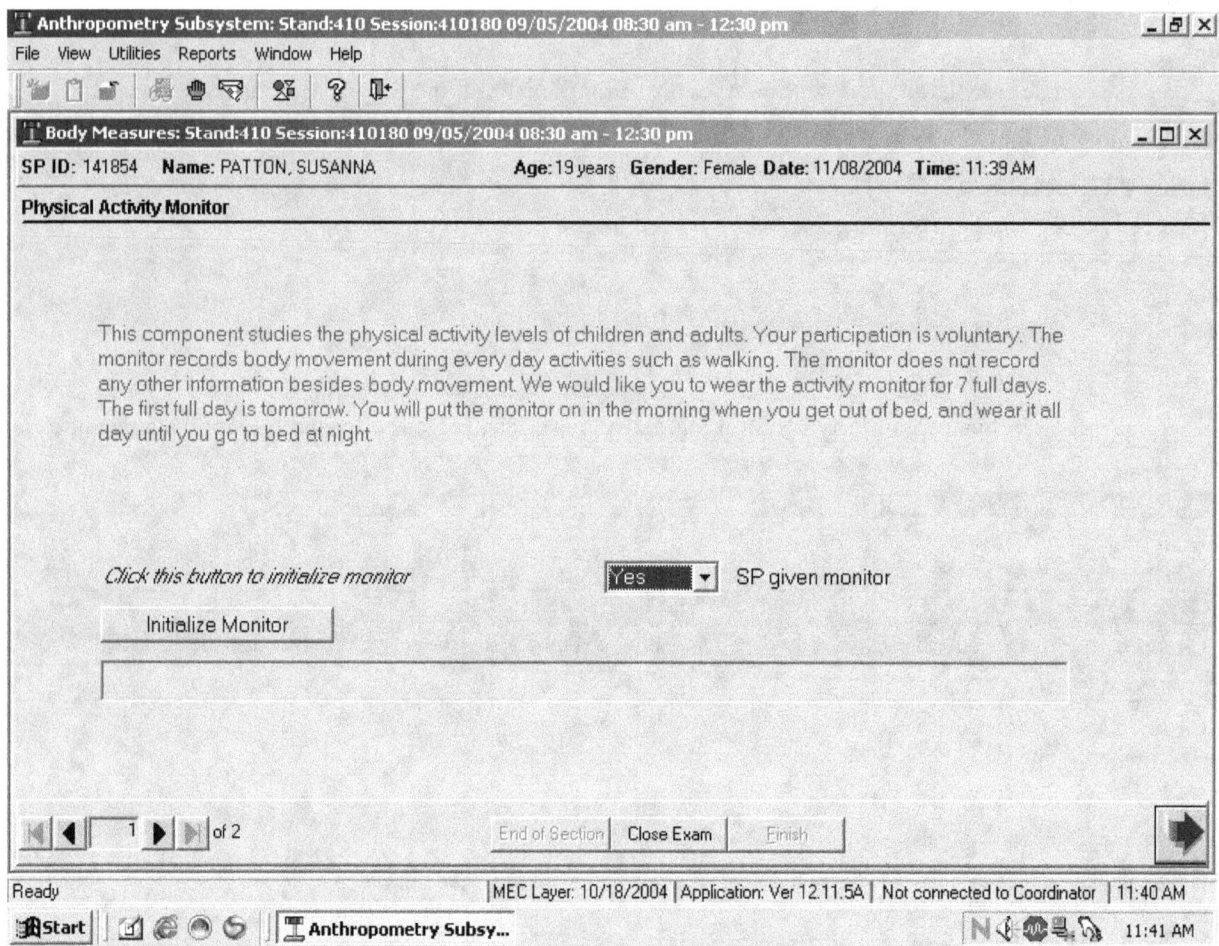

The Physical Activity Monitor slide includes a script, an Initialize Monitor button, an SP given monitor drop-down list, and a blank progress bar. Read the script as displayed. Additional talking points are displayed on the wall-mounted summary script. Use the following summary scripts (Exhibits 6-2 and 6-3) to reinforce the important points.

Exhibit 6-2. PAM script – English

## Physical Activity Monitor

- This component studies the physical activity levels of children and adults;

- The monitor records body movement during everyday activities such as walking;

- Your participation is voluntary;

- The monitor runs on a watch battery, is safe, and will not cause discomfort when worn;

- Wear the monitor all day, every day, for 7 days except when you shower, bathe, or go swimming;

- Put the monitor on when you get up in the morning and take it off before you go to bed;

- Your first full day wearing the monitor is tomorrow, however we would like you to start wearing the monitor when you get dressed before leaving here today;

- The monitor is worn on a belt. I will place the monitor on the belt and fit the belt on you;

- It is best to keep the monitor fastened on the belt to reduce the chance of losing it;

- Mail the monitor back to our home office at the end of the 7-day period;

- Place the monitor in the postage-paid padded envelope and drop the envelope in any United States Postal Service mailbox as soon as possible;

- Please do not return the belt;

- When we receive the monitor we will mail you a check for $40;

- If the monitor is not returned you will not be paid;

- Two copies of an information letter about the study are included. These are included in case you need to provide schools, camps, or work offices with information about the study;

- When passing through metal detectors at airports and work sites, it would be best to remove the monitor and put it in a separate bin for scanning. If questioned about the monitor, please show the information letter to security personnel; and

- If you have questions, please call our office using the toll-free number that is listed on the bottom of the information and instruction sheets.

Exhibit 6-3. PAM script – Spanish

## Monitor de Actividad Física

- Este componente estudia los niveles de actividad física de niños y adultos;

- El monitor registra los movimientos del cuerpo durante actividades diarias, tal como caminar;

- Su participación es voluntaria;

- El monitor funciona con una pila de reloj, es seguro y no le causará incomodidad mientras lo lleva;

- Use el monitor todo el día, todos los días por 7 días excepto cuando se ducha, se baña, o va a nadar;

- Póngase el monitor cuando se levanta en la mañana y quíteselo antes de acostarse;

- Su primer día completo para llevar el monitor es mañana, sin embargo quisiéramos que empezara a llevar el monitor cuando se vista antes de irse hoy de aquí;

- El monitor se lleva con un cinturón. Pondré el monitor en el cinturón y le ajustaré el cinturón;

- Es mejor llevar el monitor abrochado al cinturón para reducir la posibilidad de perderlo;

- Mande por correo el monitor a nuestra oficina al fin del período de 7 días;

- Ponga el monitor en el sobre abullonado con porte prepagado que le dieron y ponga el sobre en cualquier buzón del Servicio Postal de Estados Unidos lo antes posible;

- Por favor no devuelva el cinturón;

- Cuando recibamos el monitor le mandaremos un cheque por $40;

- Si no devuelve el monitor no se le pagará;

- Hemos incluido dos copias de una carta informativa acerca del estudio. Estas se incluyen en caso de que usted necesite proporcionar información acerca del estudio a escuelas, campamentos, u oficinas de trabajo;

- Cuando pase por un detector de metales en aeropuertos y lugares de trabajo, lo mejor será que se quite el monitor y lo ponga en un recipiente para que lo pasen por el escáner. Si le preguntan acerca del monitor, por favor muestre la carta informativa al personal de seguridad; and

- Si desea hacer alguna pregunta, por favor llame a nuestra oficina usando el número gratis que está anotado en la parte de abajo de las hojas informativas y de instrucción.

## 6.8      Complete the PAM Section of the Phlebotomy Exam

The activity monitor interfaces with a computer using a reader interface unit (RIU) connected to the computer in the phlebotomy room. Once the SP has agreed to participate, the health technologist puts the monitor in the RIU cradle and selects the initialization button. The activity monitor must be placed correctly in the RIU cradle in order for the monitor to be initialized. The activity monitor should be placed with the back cover and screws facing up. The notched end of the activity monitor should be directly over the finger access slot in the front wall of the RIU. When initializing and downloading make sure the PAM is inserted properly into the RIU; the light emitting diode (LED) should be visible when the PAM is inserted correctly. The flashes of the LED are observable as a reflection in the mirrored surface located in the ejection port of the RIU. To extend battery life, remove the PAM from the RIU after completing the initialization or data download.

There are three messages the health technologist may see while initializing. The first comes up if the monitor has already been initialized during the session. The program will not allow the same monitor to be initialized twice in a session. The second potential message appears if the monitor is not seated in the cradle correctly. It displays a message that indicates that it cannot read the serial number. This last message informs the health technologist the initialization is complete. If there are no problems with the initialization, this is the only message the health technologist will see. One additional popup window flashes on the screen. It indicates that the application is creating the Pf_appt (phone followup appointment). Do not press the Initialize button again.

If the SP agrees to participate and the monitor initializes successfully, the section status is Complete. If the SP is excluded or declines (refuses) to participate, then select "no" from the SP given monitor drop-down list; the section status is Not Done. Select and record the appropriate the comment for this Not Done section status.

### 6.8.1 Initialize the Monitor

If the SP is eligible for the PAMC, then the Physical Activity Monitor (initialization) slide will display after the body measures status slide.

Visually inspect the monitor. Read the script and introduce the SP to the component. To initialize the device, place the PAM in the RIU with the screws facing up and the notched end over the finger access slot in the front of the unit.

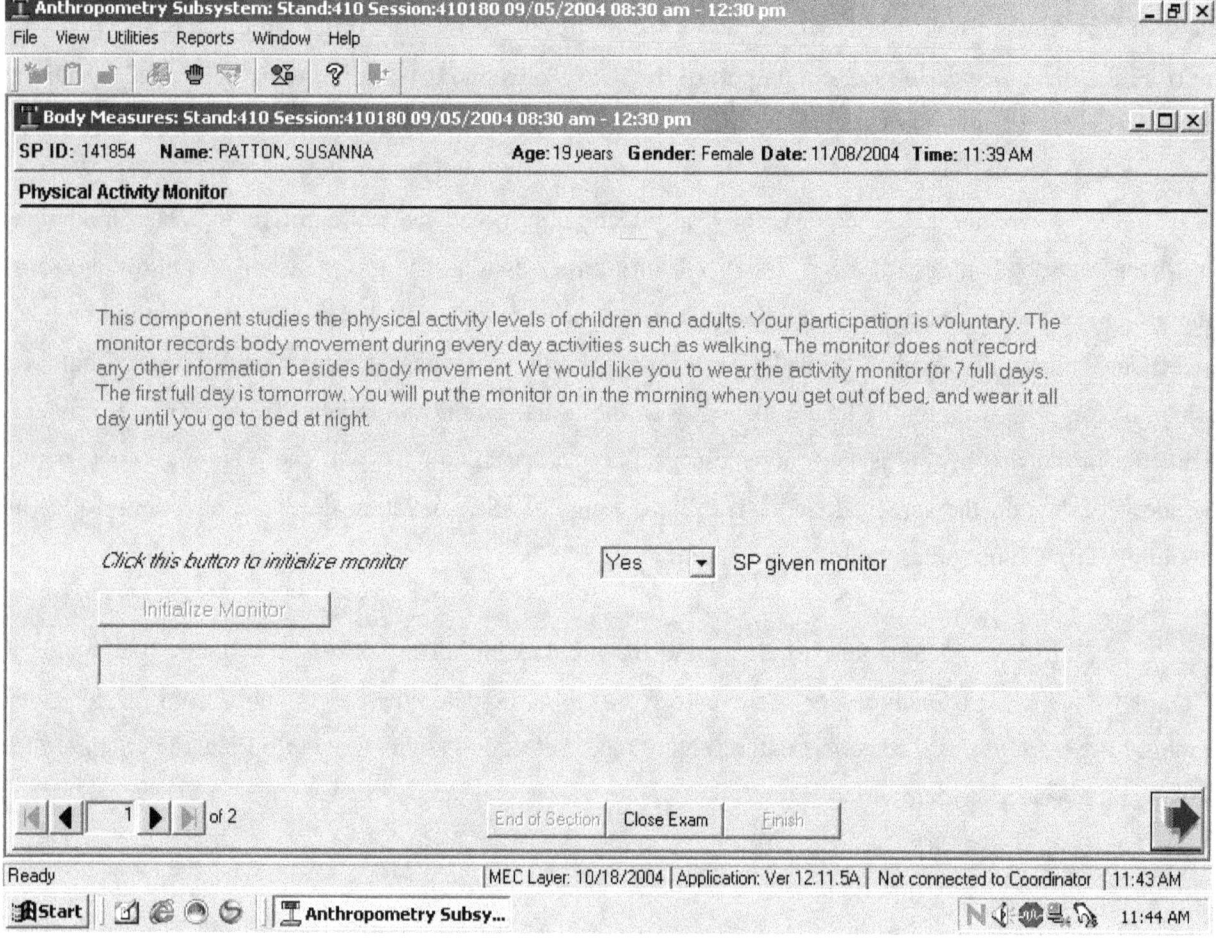

To initialize the PAM, use the mouse to direct the mouse arrow to the Initialize Monitor button and left click. The RIU may or may not display a series a red flashes as the monitor is being initialized. The Initialize Monitor button will gray out while the monitor is being initialized.

The read-only progress bar displays the initialization steps.

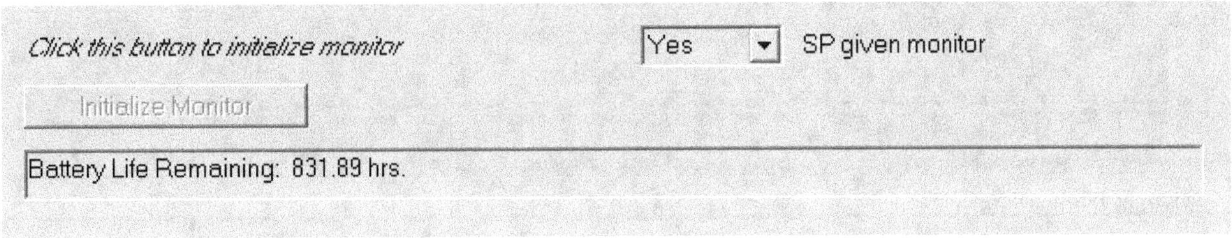

Click this button to initialize monitor    Yes  ▼   SP given monitor

Initialize Monitor

Battery Life Remaining: 831.89 hrs.

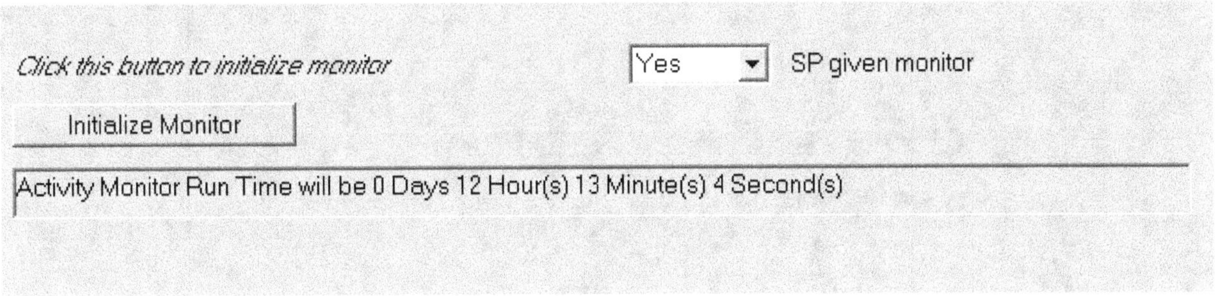

Click this button to initialize monitor    Yes  ▼   SP given monitor

Initialize Monitor

Activity Monitor Run Time will be 0 Days 12 Hour(s) 13 Minute(s) 4 Second(s)

The Battery Life Remaining and the Activity Monitor Run Time cycle through the progress bar.

If the initialization is unsuccessful, a warning message displays.

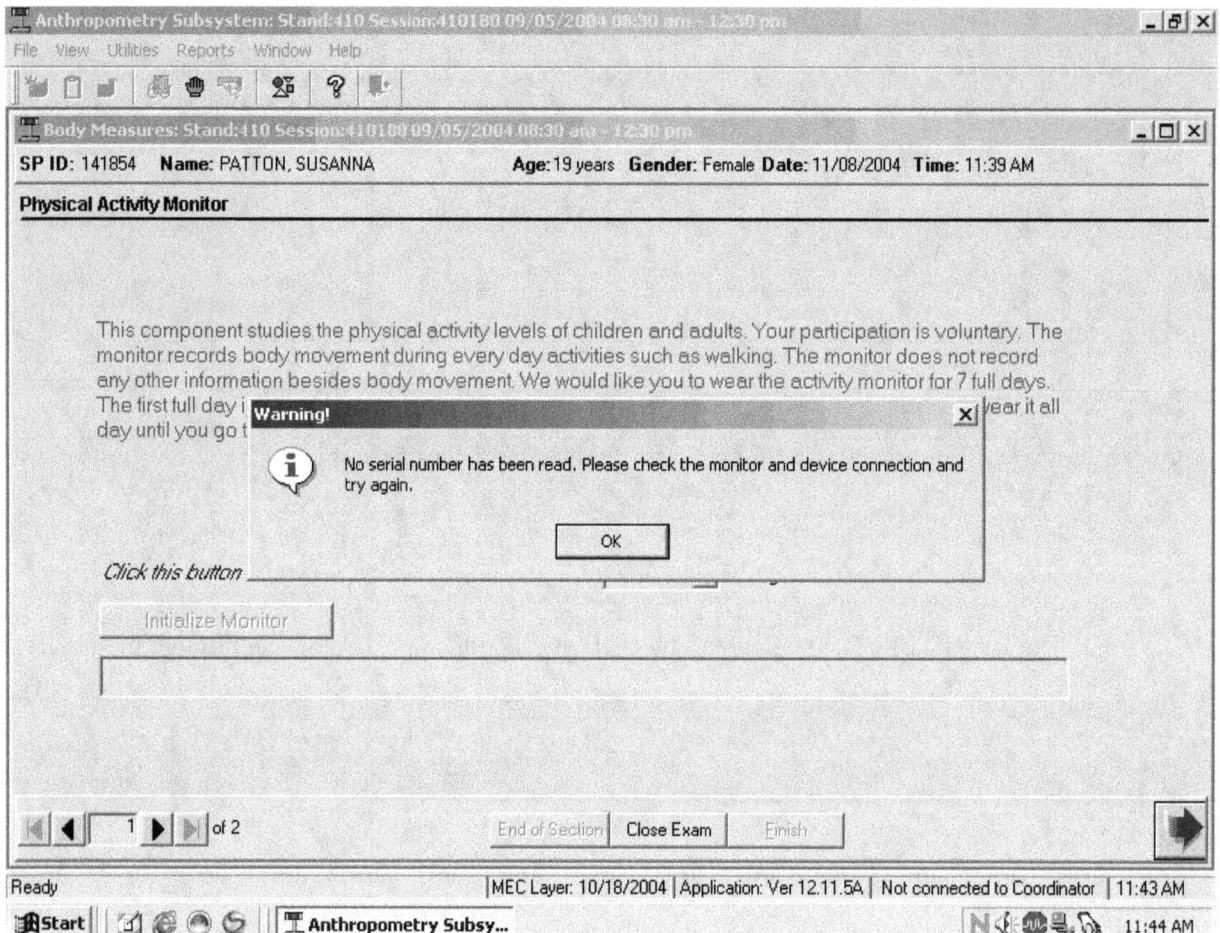

Review the message in the warning window and follow the instructions. To remove the warning message, use the mouse to direct the mouse arrow to the OK button and left click. Check the placement of the monitor in the RIU and select the Initialize Monitor button again. If the second attempt is unsuccessful, repeat the process with another monitor.

If the initialization is successful, an initialize informational window displays.

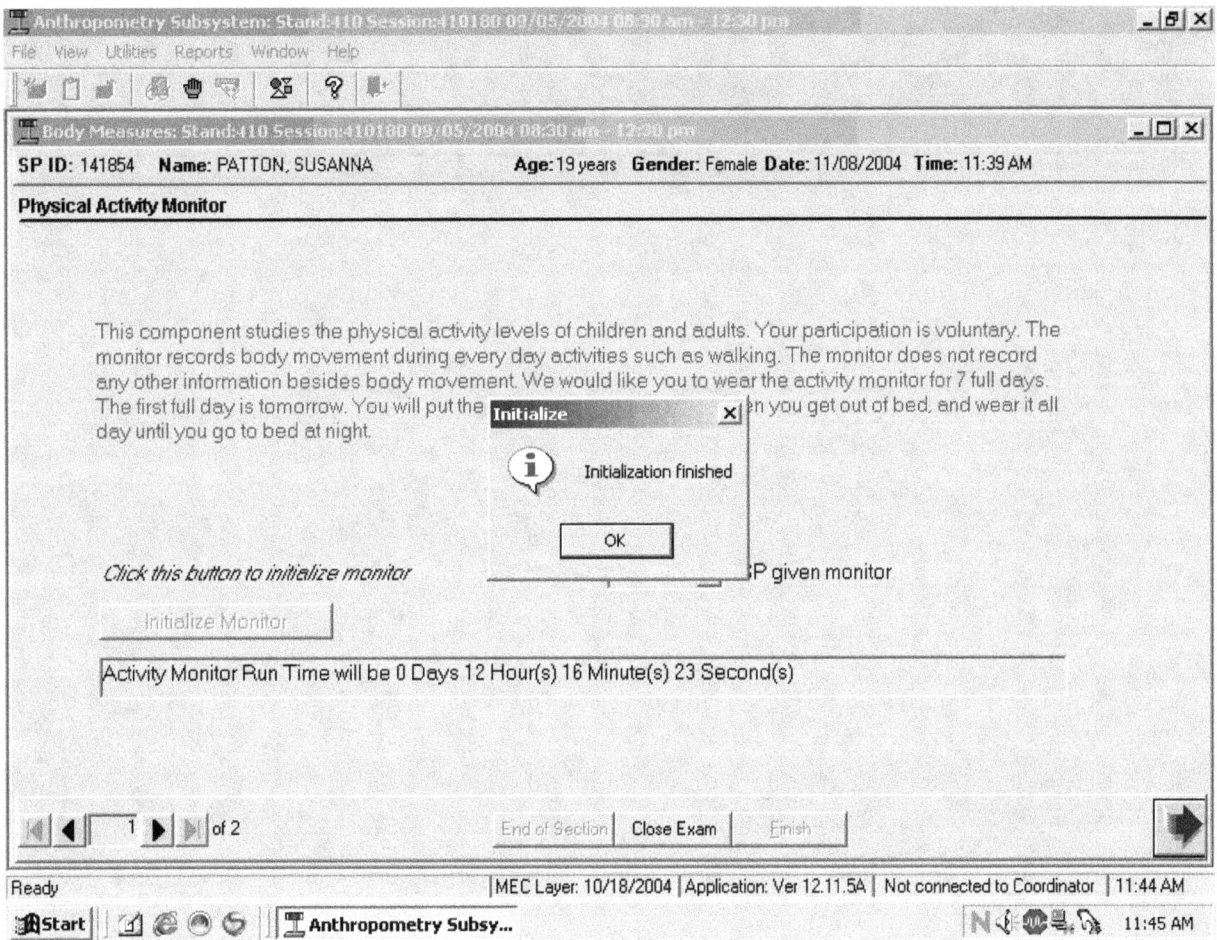

To remove the Initialize window, use the mouse to direct the mouse arrow to the OK button and left click. To move forward to the PAM section status slide, use the mouse to direct the mouse arrow to the bright blue button in the lower right hand corner and left click. Do not select [Enter] because it fires off another initialization sequence.

It is acceptable to initialize the same monitor more than once.

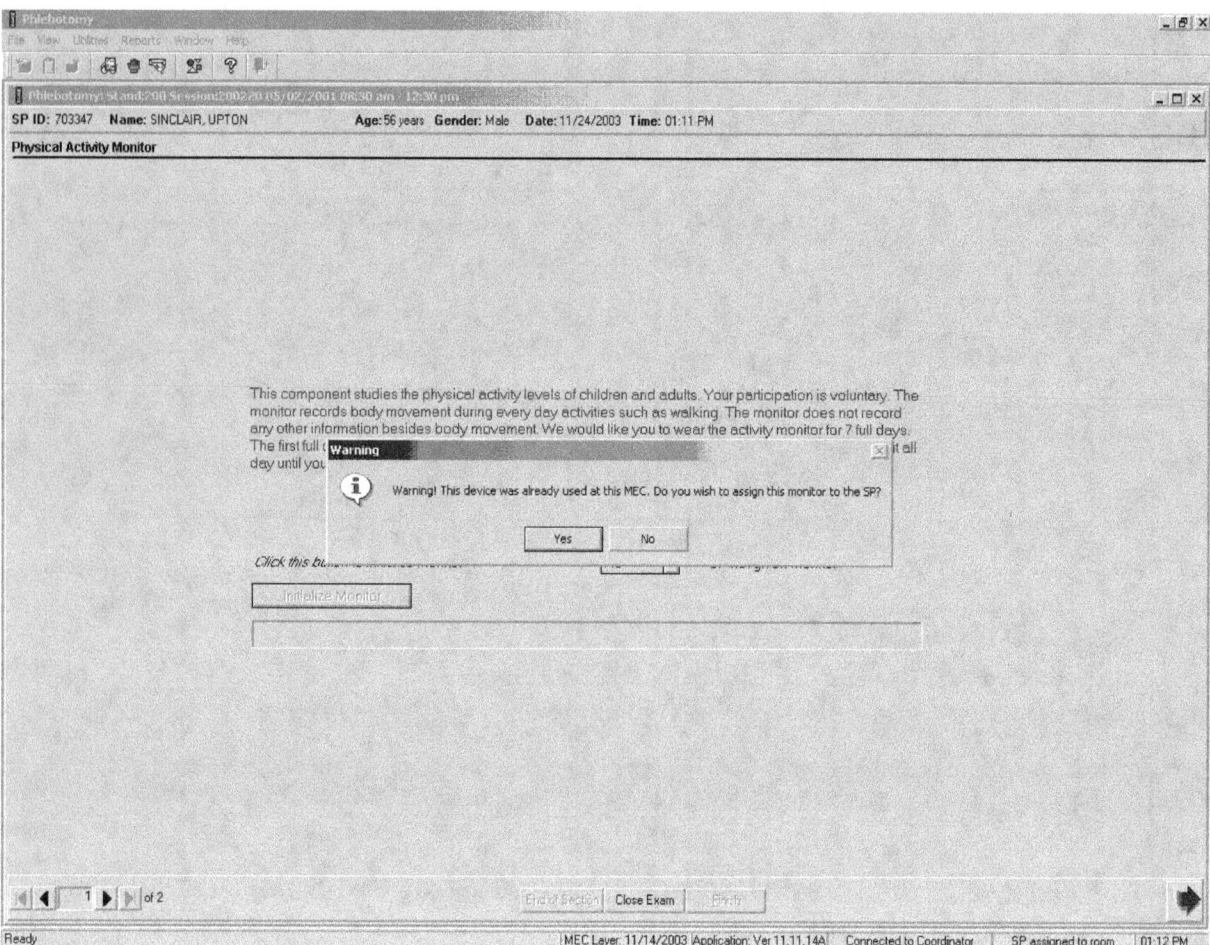

Verify that the monitor has not been assigned to another SP. To remove the warning message box and assign the monitor to the SP, use the mouse to direct the mouse arrow to the Yes button and left click or type [Enter]. To remove the warning message and skip the assignment of this monitor to this SP, use the mouse to direct the mouse arrow to the No button and left click.

It is also possible to initialize one monitor and then a second monitor for the same SP.

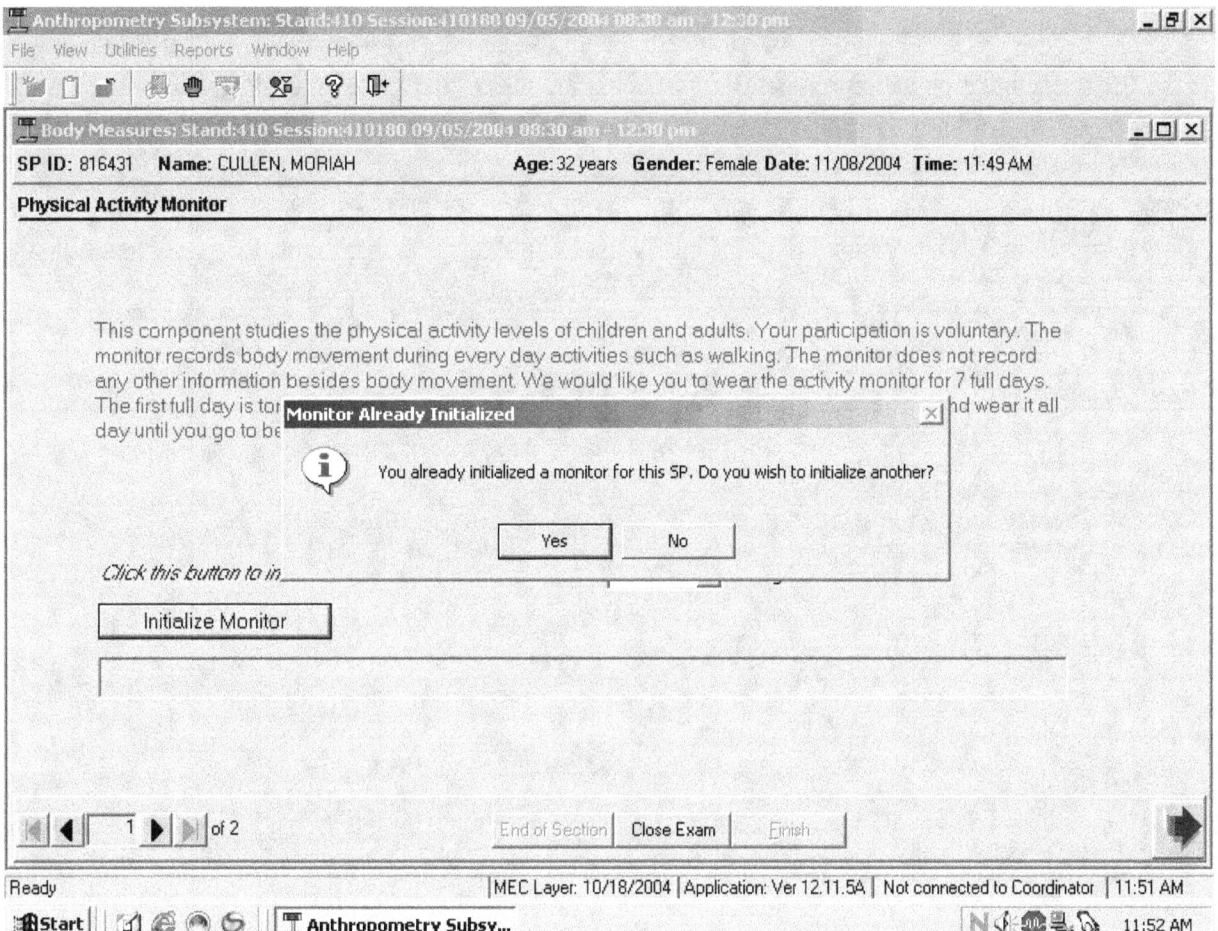

Initializing a second monitor for an SP might be required if, for example, the monitor is damaged between the time the monitor is initialized and the time the SP is exiting the MEC. It can also occur if the initialize button is accidentally hit twice. To remove the warning message box and assign the monitor to the SP, use the mouse to direct the mouse arrow to the Yes button and left click or type [Enter]. To remove the warning message and skip the assignment of this monitor to this SP, use the mouse to direct the mouse arrow to the No button and left click.

Once the monitor has been initialized, the Intermec printer in the body measures room prints one bar-coded label. The label contains an up directional arrow, the SP's name, and a bar code. Place the label on the back (side with the screws) of the monitor with the arrow pointed toward the notched end of the monitor.

### 6.8.2    SP Given Monitor

The 'SP given monitor' text box will default to "Yes," indicating that the SP is not excluded. If the SP is excluded or the recruitment is unsuccessful, select "No" from the SP given monitor drop-down list.

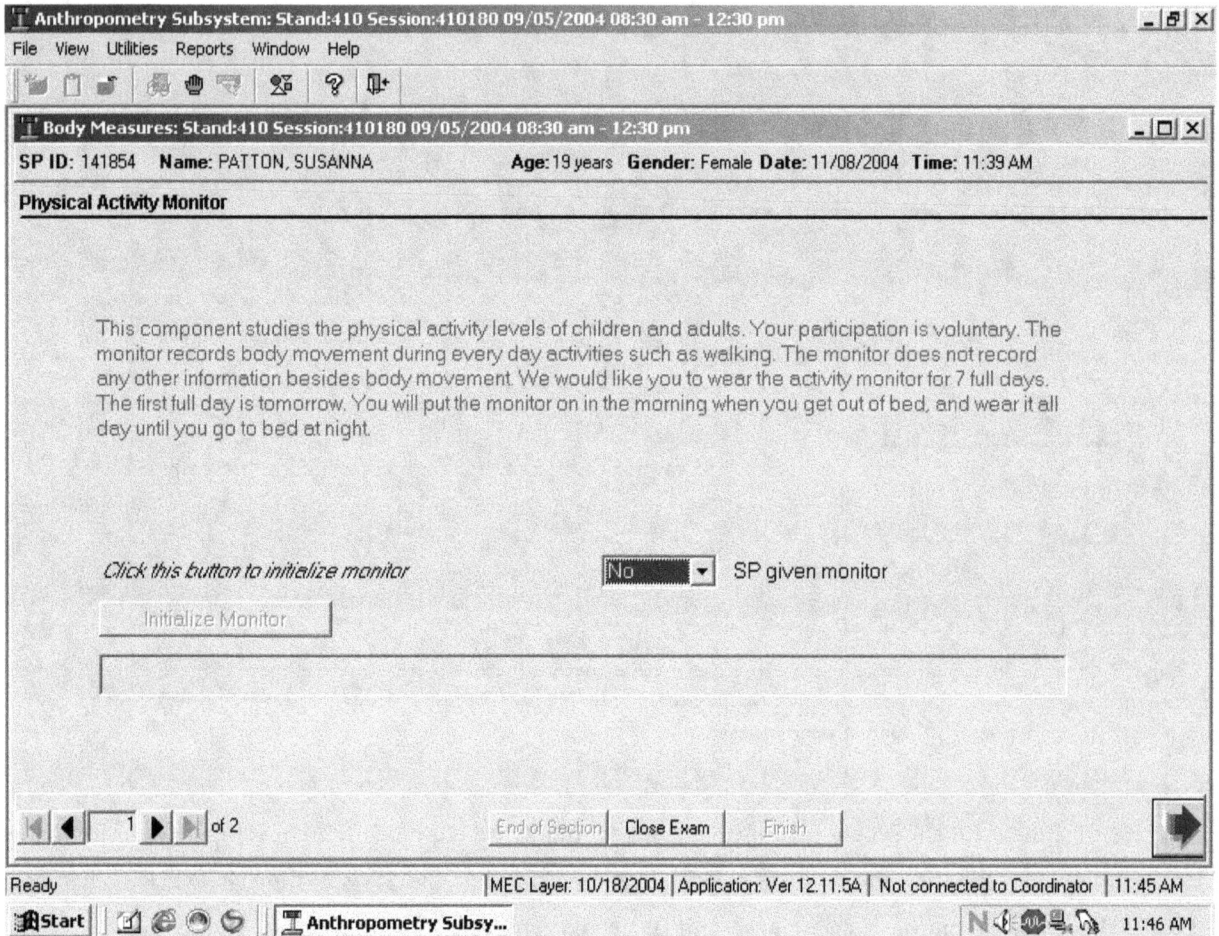

To record "No" in the SP not given monitor text box, use the mouse to direct the mouse arrow to the drop-down list, drag the arrow to "No," and left click or type [N/n]. To move forward to the PAM section status slide, use the mouse to direct the mouse arrow to the bright blue button in the lower right hand corner and left click or select [Enter].

### 6.8.3    Section Status

Review the section status slide for SPs who agree to participate.

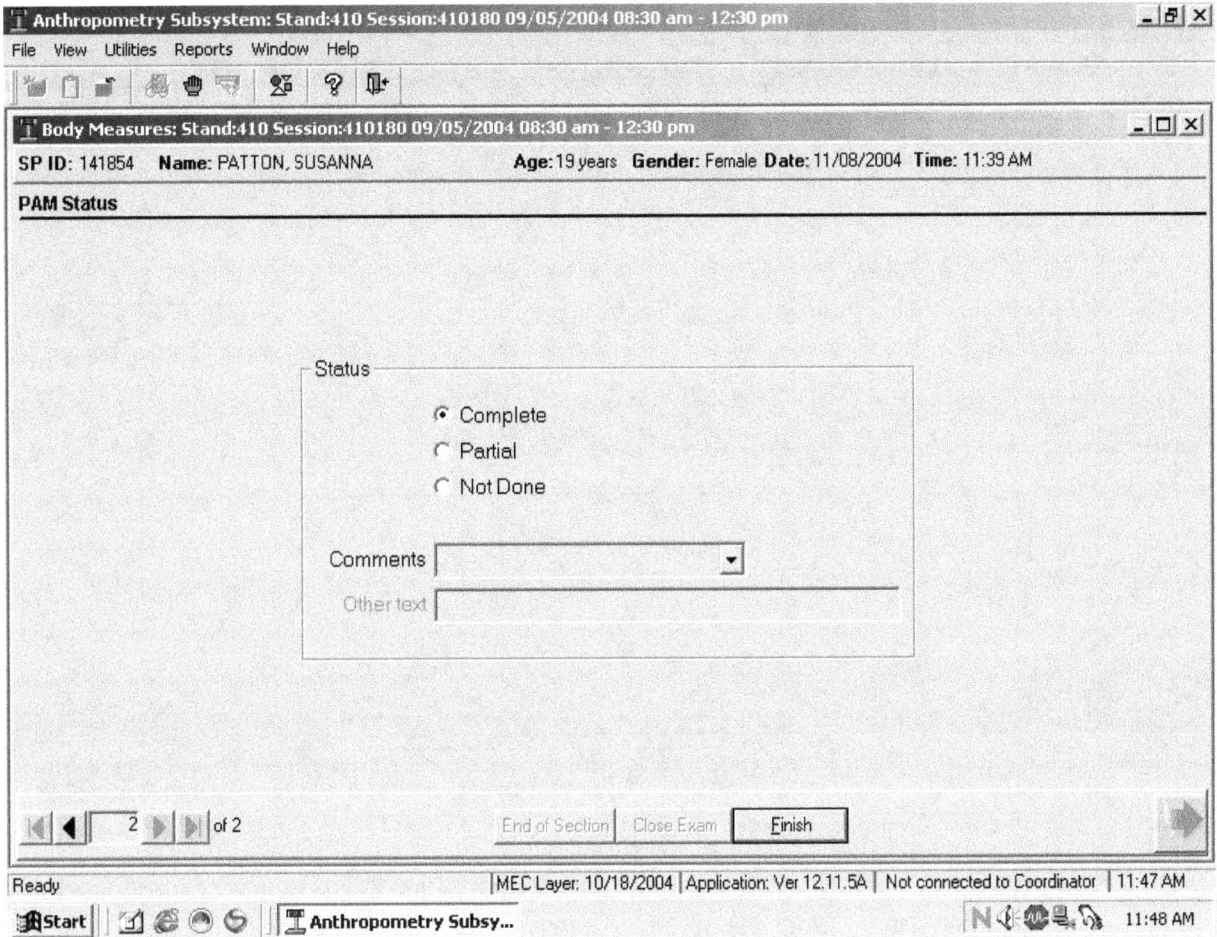

The section status is Complete if the SP agrees to participate and the monitor is successfully initialized. To complete the PAM section of the body measures exam, use the mouse to direct the mouse arrow to the Finish button in the navigation bar and left click or press [Enter] when the Finish button is highlighted.

Review the section status slide for SPs who are excluded or who do not agree to participate.

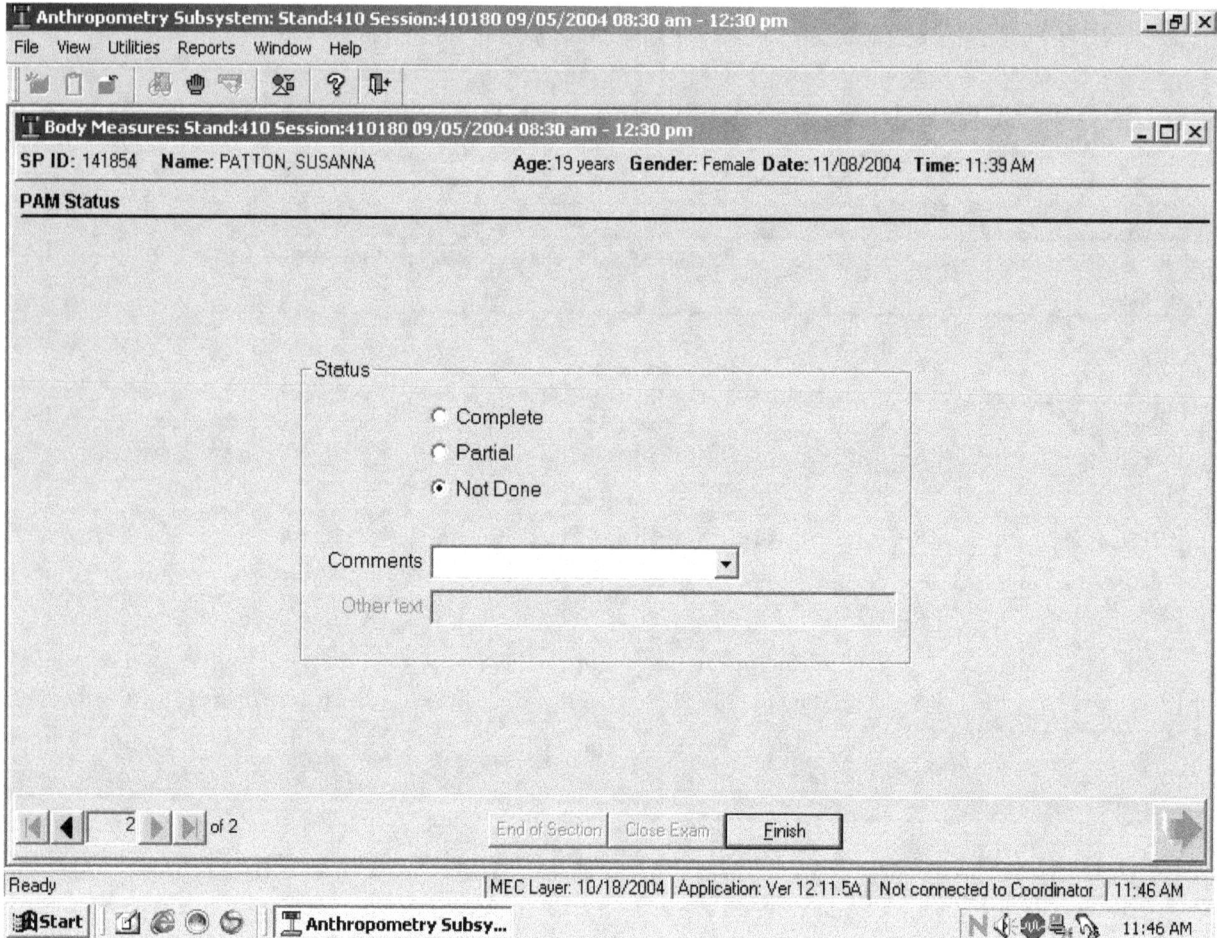

The section status is Not Done if "No" is entered in the 'SP given monitor' text box.

Choose and enter the appropriate comment code when the section status is Not Done.

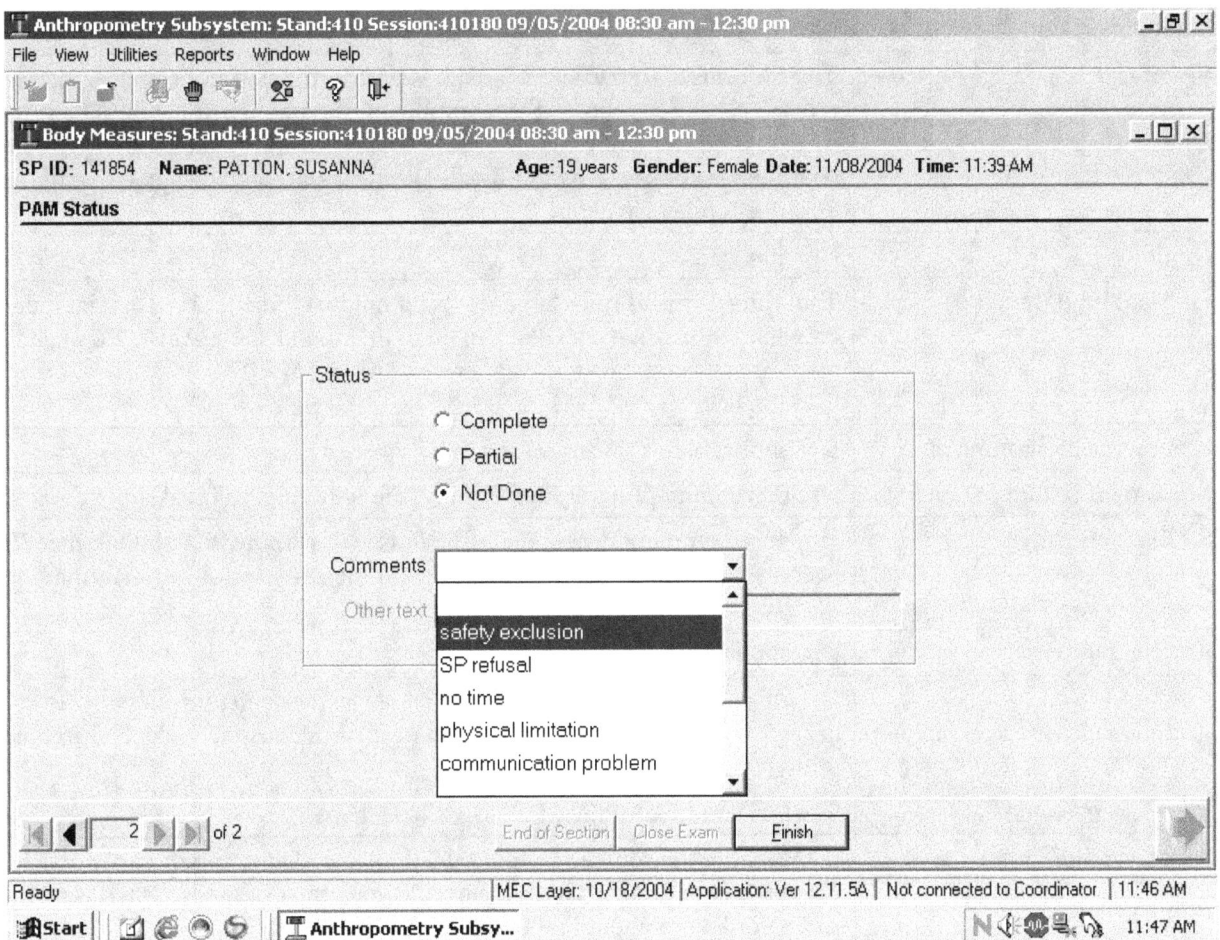

To select a comment, use the mouse to direct the mouse arrow to the drop-down list, click to display the codes, drag the arrow to select or highlight the most appropriate choice and left click. Alternatively, to select a comment code, use the up and down keyboard arrows to scroll through the choices or type the first letter of the desired comment code and when the correct choice is highlighted, left click. If "Other, specify" is chosen, type a short explanation in the "Other text" text box.

| Comment code | Use when: |
|---|---|
| Safety exclusion | The SP had recent abdominal surgery. |
| SP refusal | The SP refuses to participate. This is an SP initiated nonresponse due to refusal. The SP refuses the component for any reason other than an illness or emergency. If the SP refuses in the reception area, the coordinator codes the exam. If the SP refuses after starting the exam, the examiner codes the exam. |
| No time | Not applicable |
| Physical limitation | The SP's girth is too large to accommodate the belt. This includes pregnant SPs when the belt will not fit around their waist. Pregnancy alone is not an exclusion. SPs are excluded only if their waist is larger than the belt. |
| Communication problem | Not applicable |
| Equipment failure | Use this comment if the Reader Interface Unit fails or breaks. |
| SP ill/emergency | Use this comment when the SP faints or is about to faint or the SP becomes ill or an emergency occurs and the test cannot be performed on the SP. |
| Interrupted | Not applicable |
| Error (technician/software/supply | Use this comment when there are health technologist errors or software or supply issues. Document the event in the Unusual Field Occurrence utility. |
| Wheelchair bound | Use this comment if the SP is in a wheelchair. |
| Other, specify | If the above reason for a status Code of Not Done is not explained by one of the Comment Codes, the examiner must choose Other, specify and record a comment in the text field. |

To complete the PAM section of the body measures exam, use the mouse to direct the mouse arrow to the Finish button in the navigation bar and left click or press [Enter] when the Finish button is highlighted.

## 6.9 Fitting, Wearing, and Returning the Monitor

Place the Intermec label on the monitor, the monitor on the belt, and fit the belt on the SP. It is acceptable to place the belt and monitor on the top of a lumbar support (girdle) and on the left side as long as the monitor will not be damaged during routine wear. Keep a placebo monitor on a belt in the room as a demo and visual aid.

The information sheet has a toll-free number for the SP to call if he or she has questions. The information sheet is printed on light green paper and has English text on one side and a Spanish translation on the other. Each SP receives one copy.

Review and give one copy of the information sheet to the SP. Calculate the last day that the SP will wear the monitor; add 8 days to the exam date since the SP wears the monitor for 7 days beginning with the first day after their MEC exam. Record this date on the first line on the information sheet.

*The last day you will wear the monitor is* _____
(Example - If the SP's MEC exam date is January 6, add 8 days and write January 13 on the line.)

Review and give two copies of the informational flyer describing the component to the SP. This information flyer has a toll-free number for SP's to call if they have questions. The informational flyer is printed on NHANES letterhead and has English text on one side and Spanish on the other. Each SP receives two copies.

Complete the following steps for each SP:

- Place the label on the monitor;

- Estimate the correct length and trim the belt before beginning to place the monitor onto the belt;

- Put the monitor on the belt with the proper side up;

- Ask the SP to stand;

- Close the curtain for privacy;

- Fit the belt with the monitor attached around the SP's waist. The belt should be buckled snuggly around the SP's waist so that the monitor rests on the **right** side of the SP's body, close to his or her right hip, and the Velcro® closure is centered. The belt and the monitor should be worn under the SP's clothing;

- Trim the belt so that 4 inches remain. Be sure to trim the correct end of the belt. Leave the "easy-peel" end intact and trim the other end;

- Calculate the last day that the SP will wear the monitor; add 8 days to the exam date since the SP wears the monitor for 7 days beginning with the first day after his or her MEC exam. Record this date on the first line on the information sheet;

- Review the information sheet and informational flyer with the SP;

- Place the monitor (on the belt) back into the padded mailer;

- Place the hard copy documents back into the padded mailer;

- Transfer the number from the SP's gown (this corresponds to his or her basket number) to the outside of the padded mailer;

- Place the mailer in the basket with the SP's street clothes;

- Instruct the SP to put the monitor/belt on when he or she changes into street clothes; and

- When the SP is ready to exit the MEC, check the placement of the monitor.

Instruct the SP to wear the monitor everyday for 7 days. The SP should put the activity monitor on as soon as he or she gets out of bed in the morning and wears it all day until he or she goes to sleep at night. The monitor should not get wet, so the SP should take the monitor off while showering, bathing, or swimming. Although no injury will be caused if the SP gets the monitor wet, it might cause the instrument to malfunction. When passing through metal detectors, the SP should remove the monitor and put it in a separate bin for scanning.

## 6.10 Final Actions and Instructions

The coordinator will let the health technologist know when the SP is ready to leave the MEC. The health technologist should check with the SP to make sure he or she puts the belt containing the monitor on his or her waist and checks the monitor placement, making sure the belt is secure around the SP's waist and that the monitor is on the SP's right hip.

Each SP should exit the exam center with the following items:

- The activity monitor (SP should put this on when getting dressed.); the health technologist should check the SP before leaving the MEC);

- The padded envelope;

- Two copies of the informational flyer on survey letterhead (Exhibits 6-4 and 6-5); and

- An information sheet (Exhibits 6-6 and 6-7).

Instruct the SP to mail the monitor back to the home office after the SP has completed the 7-day period. Instruct the SP to place the monitor into the postage-paid padded envelope, seal the envelope, and place it in any United States Postal Service mail receptacle. The SP should keep or discard the belt. If the monitor is not received at the home office 12 days after the MEC exam date, the home office will initiate a series of mail and telephone contacts to ask the SP to return the monitor.

## 6.11    SP Remuneration

Once the monitor is received at the home office, the SP will be sent a check in the mail for $40. If the monitor is not returned, the SP will not receive the $40. If the monitor is lost, it is not replaced.

**6.12       Informational Flyer – English and Spanish**

Exhibit 6-4. Informational flyer – English

The Centers for Disease Control and Prevention (CDC) conducts the National Health and Nutrition Examination Survey ("NHANES") to study the health of the U.S. population. As part of this study, a group of survey participants will wear physical activity monitors such as the one pictured here. The activity monitor records body movements during normal daily activities such as walking or jogging. The activity monitor records no other information.

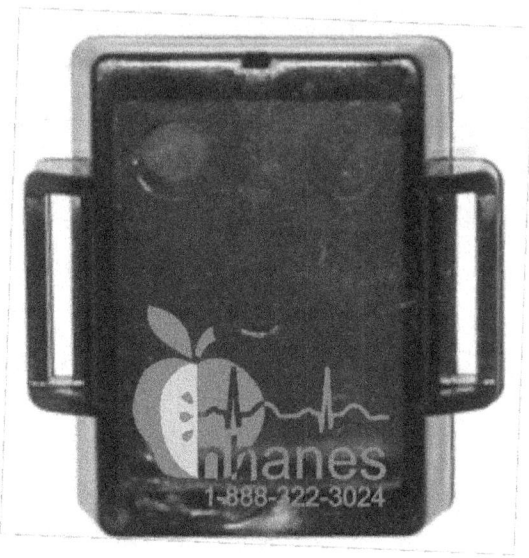

**A photograph of the NHANES Physical Activity Monitor**

Manufacturing Technology Incorporated of Fort Walton Beach, Florida manufactures the activity monitors. Over 5,000 of these monitors have been used in other studies. A 3-volt watch battery powers the monitors. The monitors are safe, durable, and comfortable to wear. The National Center for Health Statistics Institutional Review Board reviewed the survey procedures and a description of the equipment for safety.

Survey participants will wear the activity monitors for 7 days during waking hours including activities such as school, camp, or work, whenever possible. The monitors are worn on a waist belt. The monitors are removed before going to bed or when the survey participant bathes, showers, or goes swimming.

If you have additional questions please call the NHANES Survey Toll-Free Information Line Number: 1-888-322-3024.

Exhibit 6-5. Informational flyer – Spanish

Los Centros para el Control y Prevención de Enfermedades ("CDC") hacen la Encuesta Nacional de Examen de Salud y Nutrición ("NHANES") para estudiar la salud de la población de Estados Unidos. Como parte de este estudio, un grupo de participantes en la encuesta usará monitores de actividad física tal como el de esta ilustración. El monitor de actividad registra los movimientos del cuerpo durante las actividades normales tales como caminar o trotar. El monitor de actividad no registra ninguna otra información.

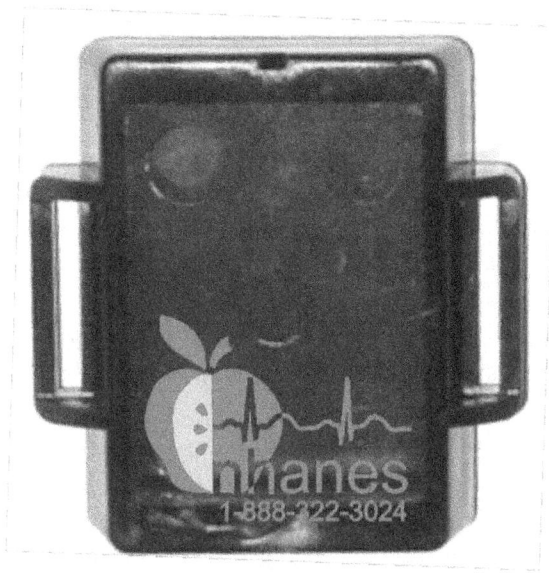

**Fotografía del Monitor de Actividad Física de NHANES**

"Manufacturing Technology Incorporated" de Fort Walton Beach, Florida fabrica los monitores de actividad. Se han usado más de 5.000 de estos monitores en otros estudios. Los monitores son seguros, durables, y cómodos de llevar. Los monitores funcionan con una pila de reloj de 3 voltios. La Junta Revisora Institucional del Centro Nacional de Estadísticas de Salud revisó la seguridad de los procedimientos de investigación y una descripción del equipo para encuestar.

Los participantes de la encuesta llevarán los monitores de actividad física por 7 días durante las horas que estén despiertos, incluyendo actividades tales como la escuela, campamento o trabajo, cuando sea posible. El monitor se lleva con un cinturón. El monitor se quita antes de acostarse o cuando el participante se baña, se ducha, o va a nadar.

Si desea hacer preguntas adicionales por favor llame al número gratis de la Línea de Información de NHANES: 1-888-322-3024.

**6.13     Information Sheet – English and Spanish**

Exhibit 6-6. Information sheet – English

**PHYSICAL ACTIVITY MONITOR INFORMATION SHEET**

*The last day you will wear the monitor is* _____

*Mail back the monitor the next day using the padded envelope that was given to you.*

**This component studies the physical activity levels of children and adults.**

➢ **What is an activity monitor?**

An activity monitor is a small machine that records information about physical activity patterns. The monitor is safe. It uses a watch battery to power the monitor. The monitor records body movement during everyday activities such as walking. The monitor is safe to wear and will not cause discomfort while you wear it. Most people forget they are wearing it because it is lightweight and small enough to fit under clothing without being seen. Many studies with children and adults have used activity monitors. We hope to learn more about the activity levels of people who participate in NHANES.

➢ **What am I supposed to do with the activity monitor?**

We ask that you wear the monitor every day for 7 days. Wear the monitor all day except when you shower, bathe, or go swimming. Your first full day wearing the monitor is tomorrow, however we would like you to start wearing the monitor when you get dressed before leaving here today. Please put the monitor on when you get up in the morning and take it off before you go to bed. Please keep the monitor away from small children and pets to avoid accidents. When the monitor is not being worn, put the monitor where children and pets cannot reach it.

➢ **How am I supposed to wear the activity monitor?**

The monitor is worn on a belt. Attach the belt snugly around your waist so that the monitor rests on the right side of your body – close to your right hip. You will ideally wear the monitor under your clothes. It is best to keep the monitor fastened on the belt to reduce the chance of losing it.

You will wear it at all times except when in the water, for instance, taking a bath or shower, or swimming. Please do not get the monitor wet. Water could damage the monitor. If you forget to take the monitor off before bathing or swimming, you will not be harmed.

➢ **What do I do after I have worn the monitor for 7 days?**

Mail the monitor back at the end of the 7-day period. Place the monitor in the postage-paid padded envelope that you were given and drop the envelope in any United States Postal Service mailbox as soon as possible. Please do not return the belt. When we receive the monitor we will mail you a check for $40. If the monitor is not returned you will not be paid.

Exhibit 6-6. Information sheet – English (continued)

➢ **What if I get questions about the monitor?**

Two copies of an information letter about the study are included. These are included in case you need to provide schools, camps, or work offices with information about the study. When passing through metal detectors at airports and work sites, it would be best to remove the monitor and put it in a separate bin for scanning. If questioned about the monitor, please show the information letter to security personnel.

➢ **Who do I contact if I have questions?**

If you have questions about the monitor, please call our office toll-free at **1-888-322-3024**.

Exhibit 6-7. Information sheet – Spanish

## HOJA DE INFORMACIÓN DEL MONITOR DE ACTIVIDAD FÍSICA

*El último día que usted usará el monitor es el* _____

*Devuelva el monitor al día siguiente usando el sobre abullonado que le dieron.*

**Este componente estudia los niveles de actividad física de los niños y de los adultos.**

➢ **¿Qué es un monitor de actividad?**

Un monitor de actividad es una pequeña máquina que registra la información acerca de patrones de actividad física. El monitor es seguro. Funciona con una pila de reloj. El monitor registra los movimientos del cuerpo durante las actividades de todos los días tal como caminar. El monitor es seguro y no le causará incomodidad mientras lo usa. La mayoría de las personas se olvidan que lo están usando porque es liviano y lo suficientemente pequeño como para usarlo debajo de la ropa sin que se vea. Muchos estudios con niños y adultos han usado monitores de actividad. Esperamos aprender más acerca de los niveles de actividad de las personas que participan en NHANES.

➢ **¿Qué debo hacer con el monitor de actividad?**

Pedimos que usted use el monitor diariamente por 7 días. Use el monitor todo el día excepto cuando se ducha, baña, o va a nadar. Su primer día completo para usar el monitor es mañana, sin embargo, quisiéramos que empezara a llevar el monitor cuando se vista antes de irse hoy de aquí. Por favor póngase el monitor cuando se levante en la mañana y quíteselo antes de acostarse. Por favor mantenga el monitor lejos del alcance de los niños y animales domésticos para evitar accidentes. Cuando no esté llevando el monitor, ponga el monitor donde los niños y los animales domésticos no puedan alcanzarlo.

➢ **¿Cómo debo llevar el monitor de actividad?**

El monitor se lleva con un cinturón. Póngase el cinturón ajustado alrededor de la cintura de modo que el monitor quede al lado derecho de su cuerpo – cerca de la cadera derecha. Lo ideal sería que llevara el monitor debajo de la ropa. <u>Lo mejor es mantener el monitor ajustado con el cinturón para reducir la posibilidad de perderlo.</u>

Usted lo llevará en todo momento excepto cuando está en el agua, por ejemplo mientras se baña o se ducha, o nada. Por favor no moje el monitor. El agua puede dañar el monitor. Si a usted se le olvida quitarse el monitor antes de bañarse o nadar, no se hará daño a usted mismo(a).

Exhibit 6-7. Information sheet – Spanish (continued)

➢ **¿Qué debo hacer después de haber llevado el monitor por 7 días?**

Devuelva por correo el monitor al fin del período de 7 días. Ponga el monitor en el sobre abullonado con porte prepagado que le dieron y ponga el sobre en cualquier buzón del Servicio Postal de Estados Unidos lo antes posible. <u>Por favor no devuelva el cinturón</u>. Cuando recibamos el monitor le mandaremos un cheque por $40. Si no devuelve el monitor no se le pagará.

➢ **¿Qué puedo hacer si alguien me pregunta acerca del monitor?**

Hemos incluido dos copias de una carta informativa acerca del estudio. Estas se incluyen en caso de que usted necesite proporcionar información acerca del estudio a escuelas, campamentos, u oficinas de trabajo. Cuando pase por un detector de metales en aeropuertos y lugares de trabajo, lo mejor será que se quite el monitor y lo ponga en un recipiente para que lo pasen por el escáner. Si le preguntan acerca del monitor, por favor muestre la carta informativa al personal de seguridad.

➢ **¿Con quién me comunico si deseo hacer alguna pregunta?**

Si desea hacer alguna pregunta acerca del monitor, por favor llame gratis a nuestra oficina al **1-888-322-3024**.

## 6.14　Home Office Responsibilities

Upon completion of the 7-day test period, survey participants mail the PAM device to the NHANES warehouse using a postage-paid padded envelope. Separate return mailing envelopes are provided for each survey participant's PAM device. Once the monitor is received at the home office, the warehouse staff download the data and clean and calibrate each monitor. The warehouse staff check the battery life and install new batteries when the remaining battery life reaches 1,000 hours. Each PAM should cycle through 10 SPs before the battery life reaches 1,000 hours.

## 6.14.1　Battery Replacement

The battery used in the activity monitor is a lithium coin cell designated in the industry as a CR2430. Battery life is typically in excess of 4,000 hours. Actual battery life is dependent on the frequency of data downloads and the capacity of the particular manufacturer's battery. The battery life remaining, as reported by the activity monitor, is an estimate and should be interpreted as such. The voltage of a lithium battery cannot be used to predict battery life. The activity monitor estimates the remaining battery life by keeping track of total hours of operation since the last battery replacement. The 4,000-hour battery life is a safe estimate of run time for a 220-mah capacity battery (typical of the CR2430 series).

If the PAM is accidentally left in the RIU for long periods (where the LED flashes constantly), then battery life will be less than the expected 4,000 hours. Collected data will **not** be lost if the battery dies while the monitor is in the field. The activity monitor stops collecting data when the battery dies. Installing a new battery will allow the data to be downloaded.

Replace the battery when the remaining battery life reaches 1,000 hours.

To replace the battery, follow these steps:

**Step 1**

- Using a small Phillips head screwdriver, carefully remove the four screws that retain the cover on the PAM. (If the screwdriver is allowed to slip in the head of the screw, damage to the screw head will occur. If this happens, send the PAM to the factory for removal of the damaged screw.)

■ After all four screws have been removed; carefully pry off the plastic cover to expose the battery and holder. It is helpful to use one of the loose screws to extract the cover. This is done by catching the threads in one of the holes and pulling away from the case. Do not attempt to remove the circuit boards from the metal box or touch the sensor. Touching the sensor, even lightly, can damage it.

## Step 2

■ Remove the battery by inserting a small common blade jeweler screwdriver between the battery and the holder. Note that this terminal position is near the sensor. Use gentle force to release the battery. This method prevents damage to the small nibs that retain the battery. Use minimal force to avoid permanently deforming the battery holder's retaining ears.

## Step 3

■ Insert a new battery into the holder by snapping it into place. The positive (+) terminal faces up. Using a conductivity object, such as a brightly finished jeweler screwdriver or a paper clip, temporarily short the new battery by bridging the gap at the same location where the battery was pried out. This action ensures proper startup of the activity monitor processor by forcing a power-on reset. Do not skip this step.

■ Ensure that the battery holder nibs are in good shape and that they will retain the battery tightly in the holder. Nibs that are worn or spread away from the battery render the holder unreliable and will require service at the factory.

## Step 4

■ Align the sealing gaskets (if used) before installing the cover. Carefully place the cover over the box. Verify that the sides of the box are facing the interior of the lid's shield. It may be easier to temporarily remove the metal box from the plastic case and place the box onto the cover.

## Step 5

■ Place the box/lid assembly into the plastic case taking care that the holes in the box are oriented towards the notch. After all the screws have been started, snug each one up very lightly while seating the cover between the thumb and forefinger.

### 6.14.2    Cleaning

The activity monitor is water-resistant but is not waterproof. Care must be taken not to immerse it into water. Remove the label after downloading the data and clean the polycarbonate case with a Sani-Wipe cloth. Soap and water or Isopropyl alcohol may be used in an emergency. Do not use cleaning solvents or immerse the case into any liquid. Chlorinated fluorocarbon cleaners will damage the plastic case.

### 6.14.3    Download the Data and Calibrate the Monitor

Open and log onto the download application. Download the data from the monitor by placing the monitor into the RIU. Access {File} and then {Open} in the top tile bar to open the data download window. Follow the instructions on the screen.

Open the application by double clicking on the Data Download application icon on the desktop. The MEC Logon window displays.

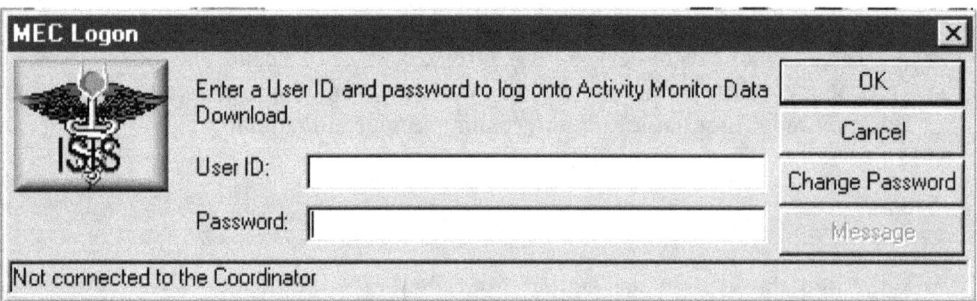

To log onto the Data Download application, type last name, underscore, first initial (Last Name_First Initial) in the User ID space, and then select [Tab] or [Enter]. Enter the password using the keyboard keys and press [Tab], [Enter], or use the mouse to direct the arrow to the OK button and left click. To exit this screen without entering a password, use the mouse to direct the arrow to the Cancel button and left click.

Open an exam.

The PAM screen displays. To open an exam, use the mouse to direct the mouse arrow to {File} in the menu bar, left click, drag the arrow to {Open} and left click, or type [Alt] [F/f], [O/o], or [Ctrl] [O/o].

The PAM Data Download window displays.

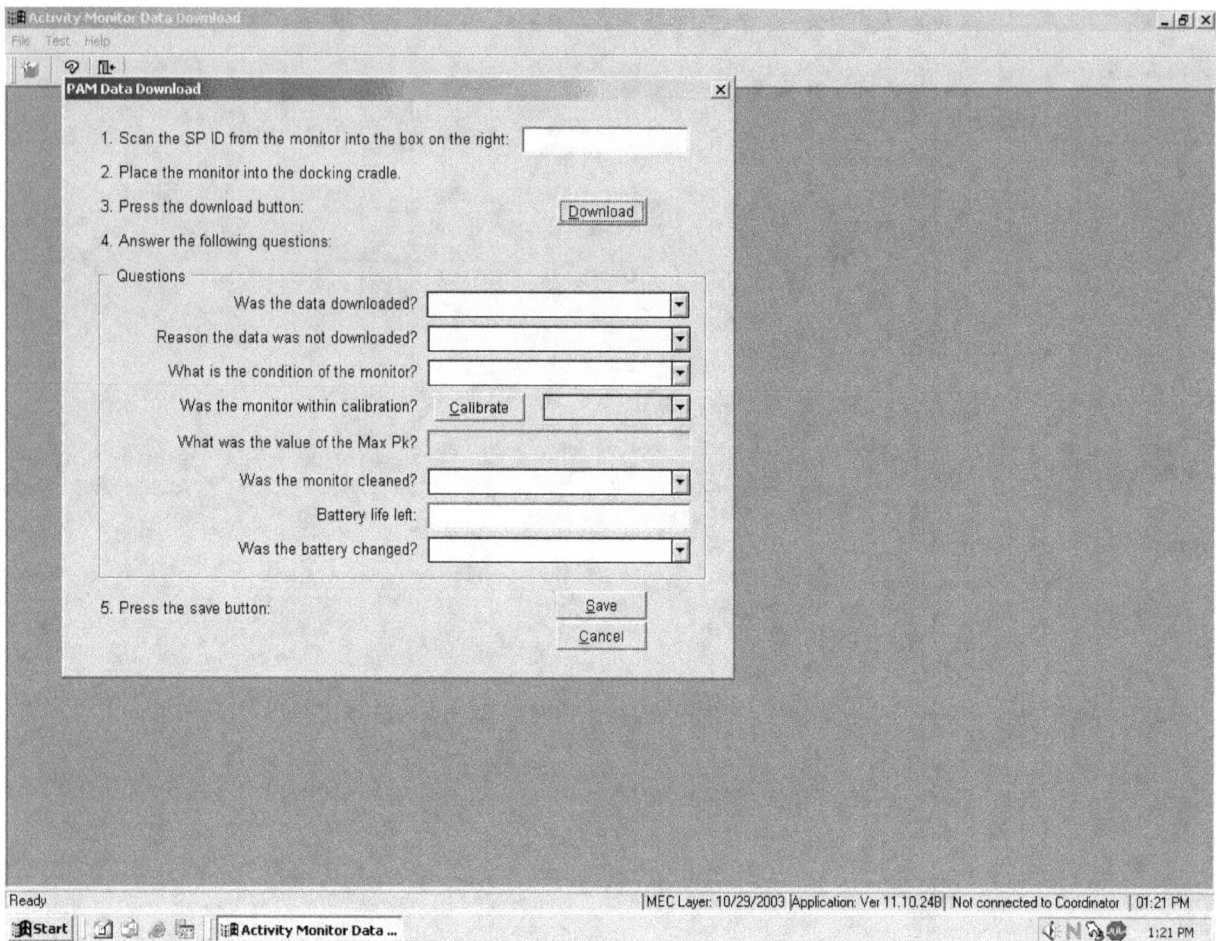

The PAM Data Download window contains a list of steps and action buttons. Scan or type the SP ID from the back of the monitor into the first text box. The application performs a validity check to verify that the SP ID matches the list of recruited SP IDs. Place the monitor into the docking cradle in the RIU with the notched side down, toward the front of the RIU and with the screws facing up. Press the Download button and observe the brown status line while the data is downloaded. Remove the monitor when the data download is complete. Answer the questions in the Questions box. If the answer to the first question, "Was the data downloaded" is "Not downloaded," then the second question is enabled.

**Calibrate the Monitor**

To calibrate a monitor:

1.  Position the calibration unit cradle with the open side facing the up position.

2.  Gently slide the monitor into the calibration cradle with the screws to the back and the smooth side toward the front and the notches down. The LED should flash red.

3.  Begin the calibration by selecting the Calibrate button. This action launches the MTI calibration program.

4.  Select the Serial Communication port number "2" when the calibration program asks for the port number.

5.  The calibration unit rotates or spins the monitor during the actual calibration.

6.  Watch the calibration graph as the monitor is calibrating.

    Evaluate the calibration data. The calibration program displays a Max Pk number after the calibration is complete. This number must be between 0.57 and 0.63.

    -   If the number is between 0.57 and 0.63 then no adjustment is necessary and the monitor is calibrated.

    -   If the number is <0.57 or >0.63, then the monitor is not in calibration and must be sent to MTI for repair.

7.  Press the [Enter] key to exit the calibration program.

Answer the next two questions and review the Battery life left number. If the battery life is less than or equal to 1,000 hours then change the battery and record this action in the last question text box. Select the Save button to save the answers to the questions and the data to the database, or select the Cancel button to repeat all of these actions, including the download.

Insert the SP ID into the text box.

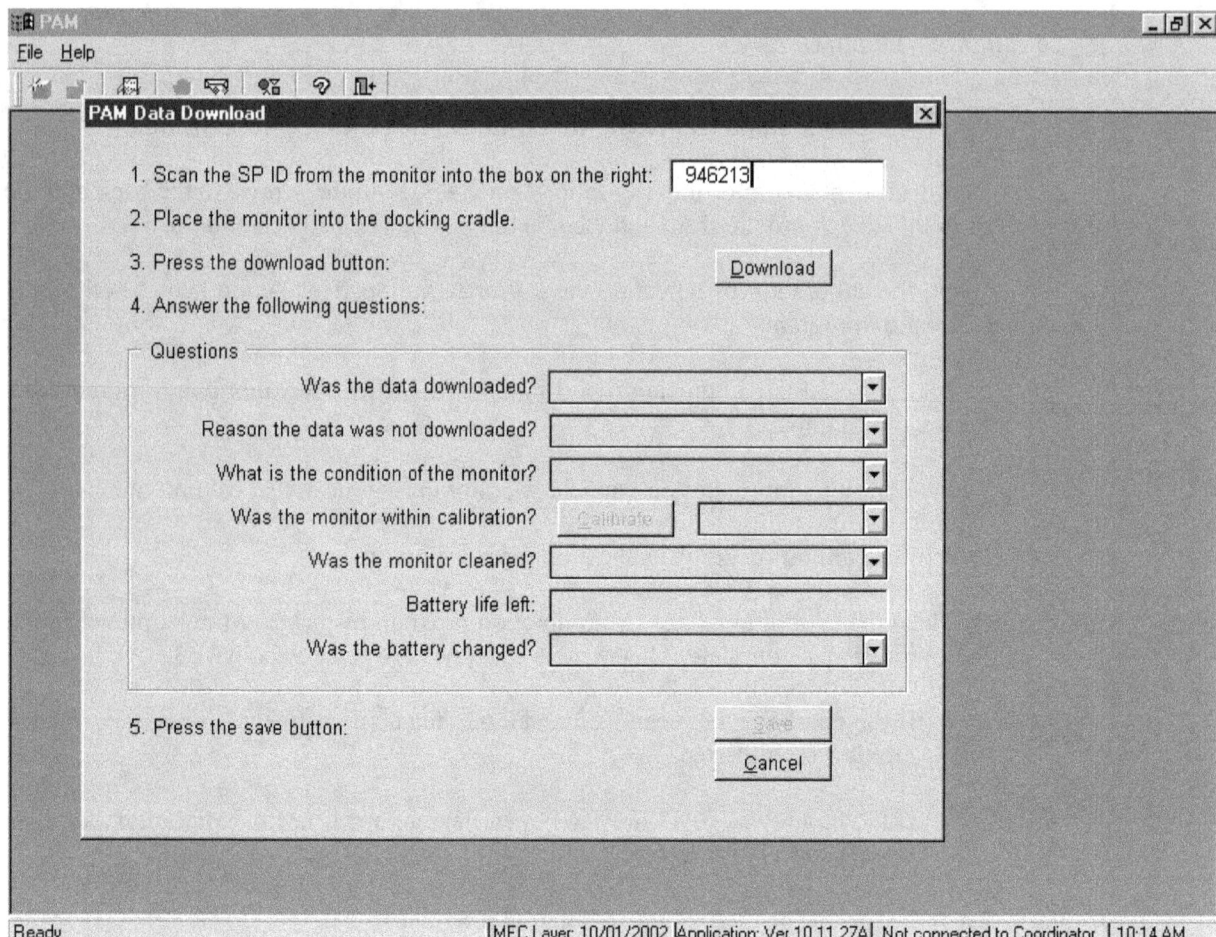

To insert the SP ID into the first text box, (Scan the SP ID from the monitor into the box on the right.) use the bar code gun to scan the bar code on the label located on the back of the monitor. Alternatively, use the keyboard numbers to type the number into the text box. If there is no label or if the label is unreadable, contact the senior system analyst. The analyst can search the database to locate the SP ID that matches the serial number that is printed on the end of the monitor case.

If the SP ID does not match a recruited SP ID, then an informational text box displays.

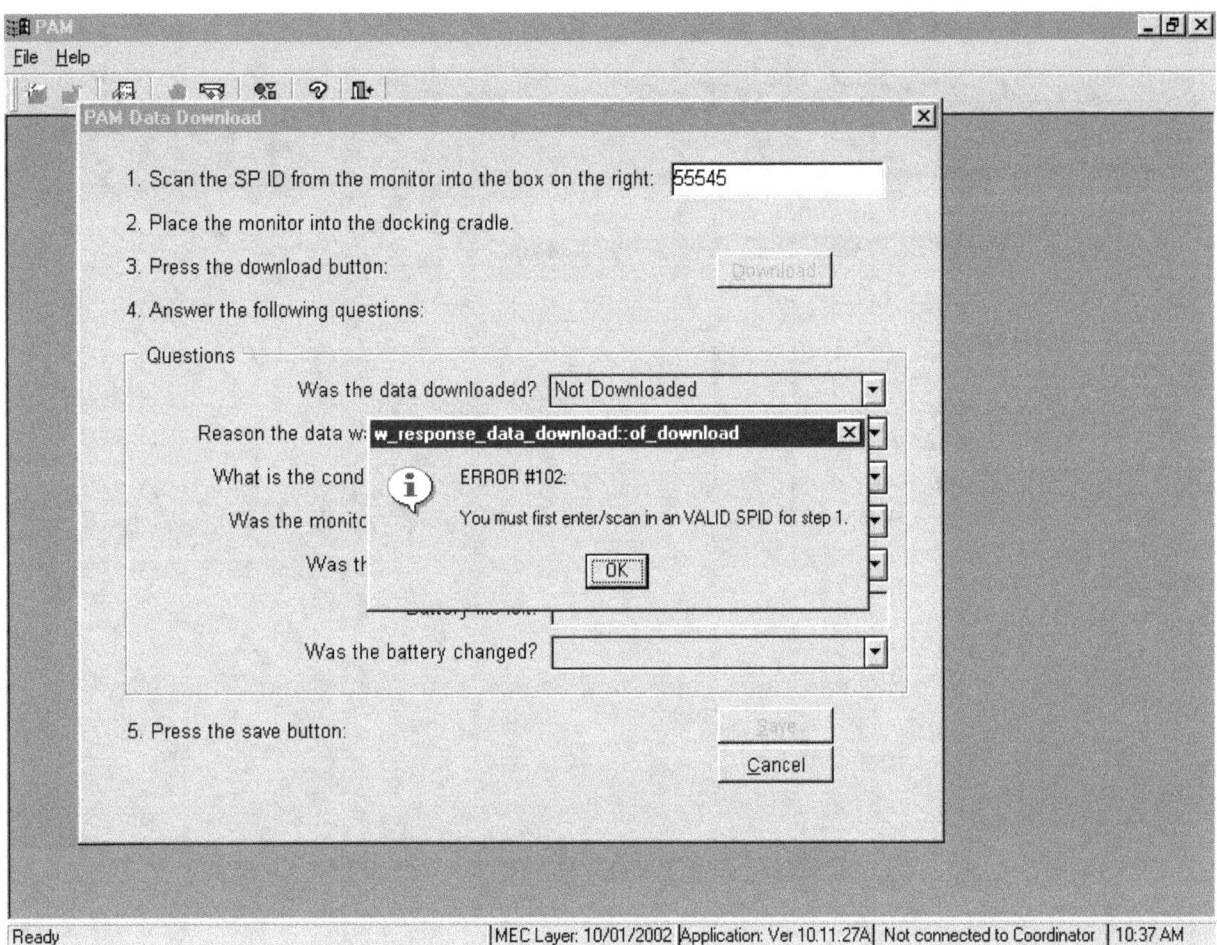

To remove the informational text box, use the mouse to direct the mouse arrow to the OK button and left click or select [Enter]. Reenter the SP ID.

Download the data.

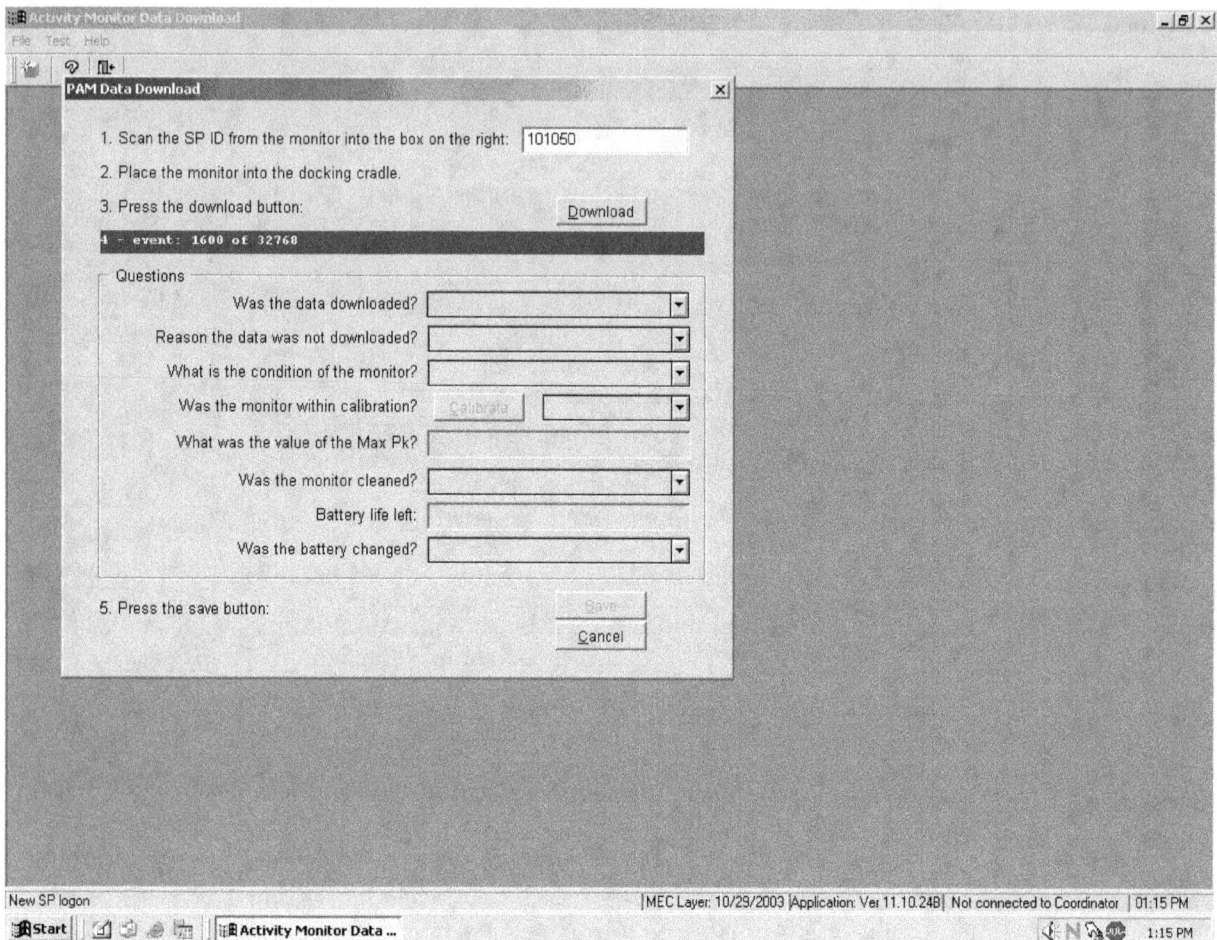

Place the monitor into the RIU docking cradle as described in Section 6.8. To begin the data download process, use the mouse to direct the mouse arrow to the Download button and left click.

Watch the brown status line while the data is downloading.

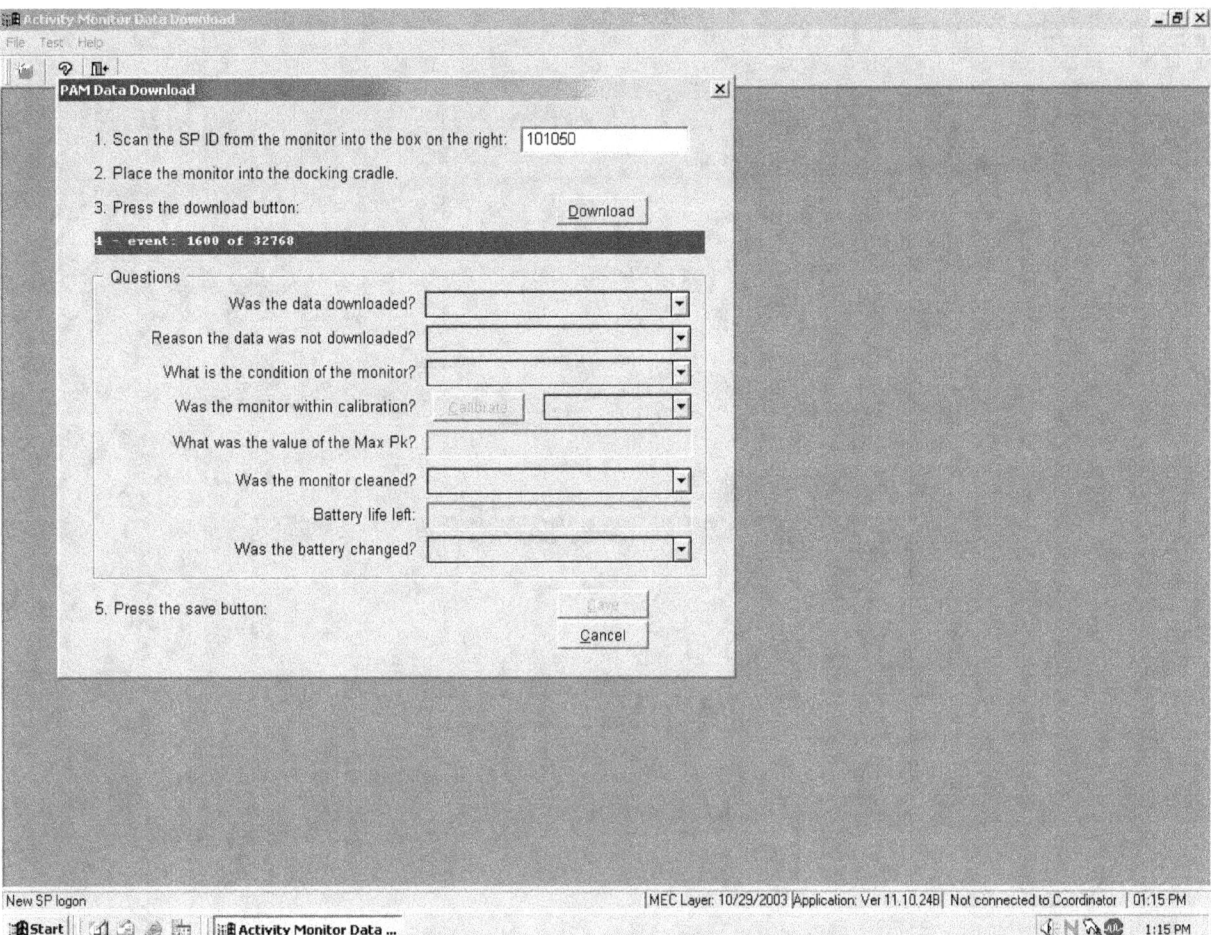

Once the Download button has been selected, a brown status line displays the various download process steps. Watch these process steps as the download progresses.

If the Download button is selected and data have already been downloaded for a SP or if the Download button is selected while the data are downloading, then an Activity Monitor Download message box displays.

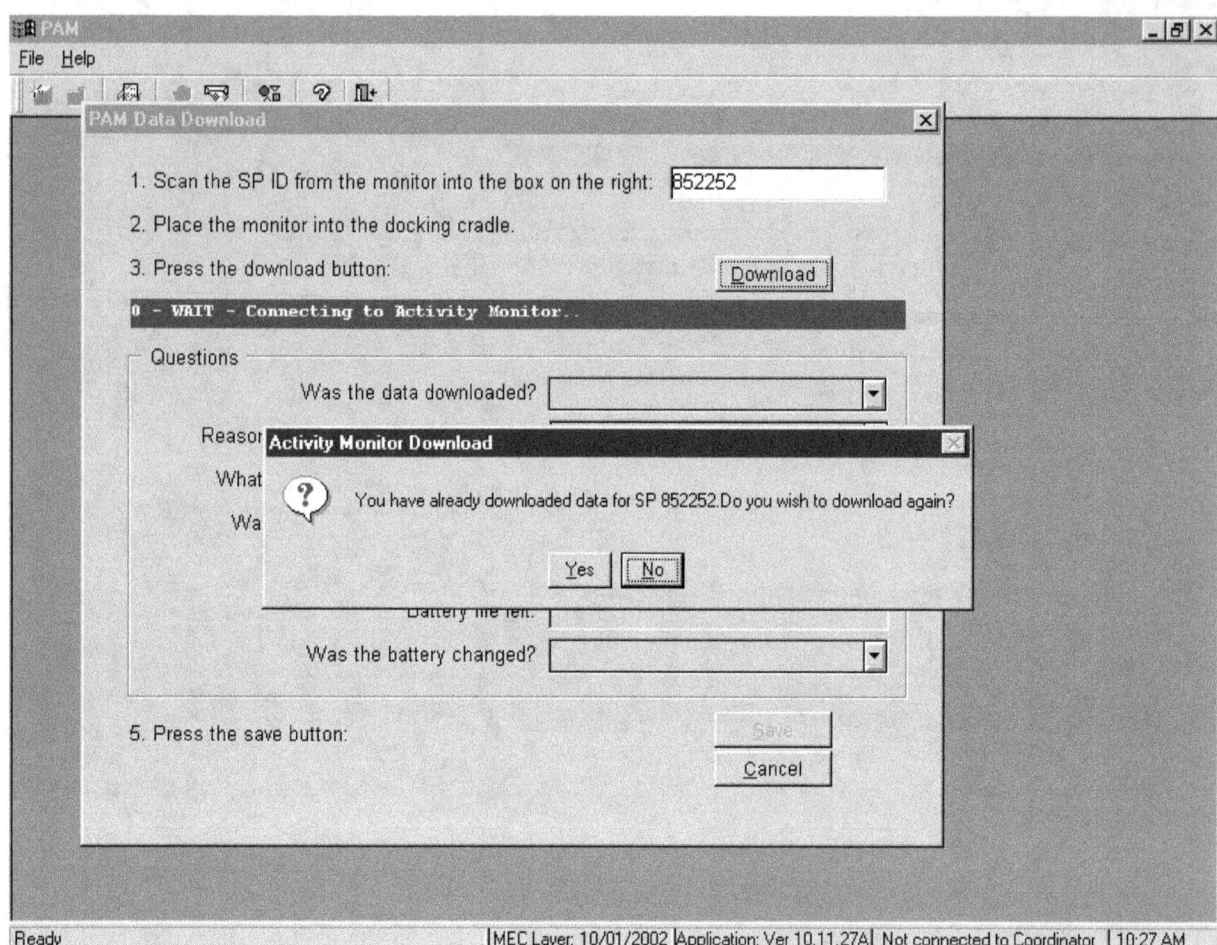

Downloading data more than once does not cause any damage to the monitor or the data in the database. To remove the message window and to download data a second time, use the mouse to direct the mouse arrow to the Yes button and left click. To cancel the additional download request, use the mouse to direct the mouse arrow to the No button and left click or select [Enter].

Once the data download is complete, the Questions in the highlighted box are activated. Remove the monitor from the RIU when the data download is complete and answer the first question, "Was the data downloaded?"

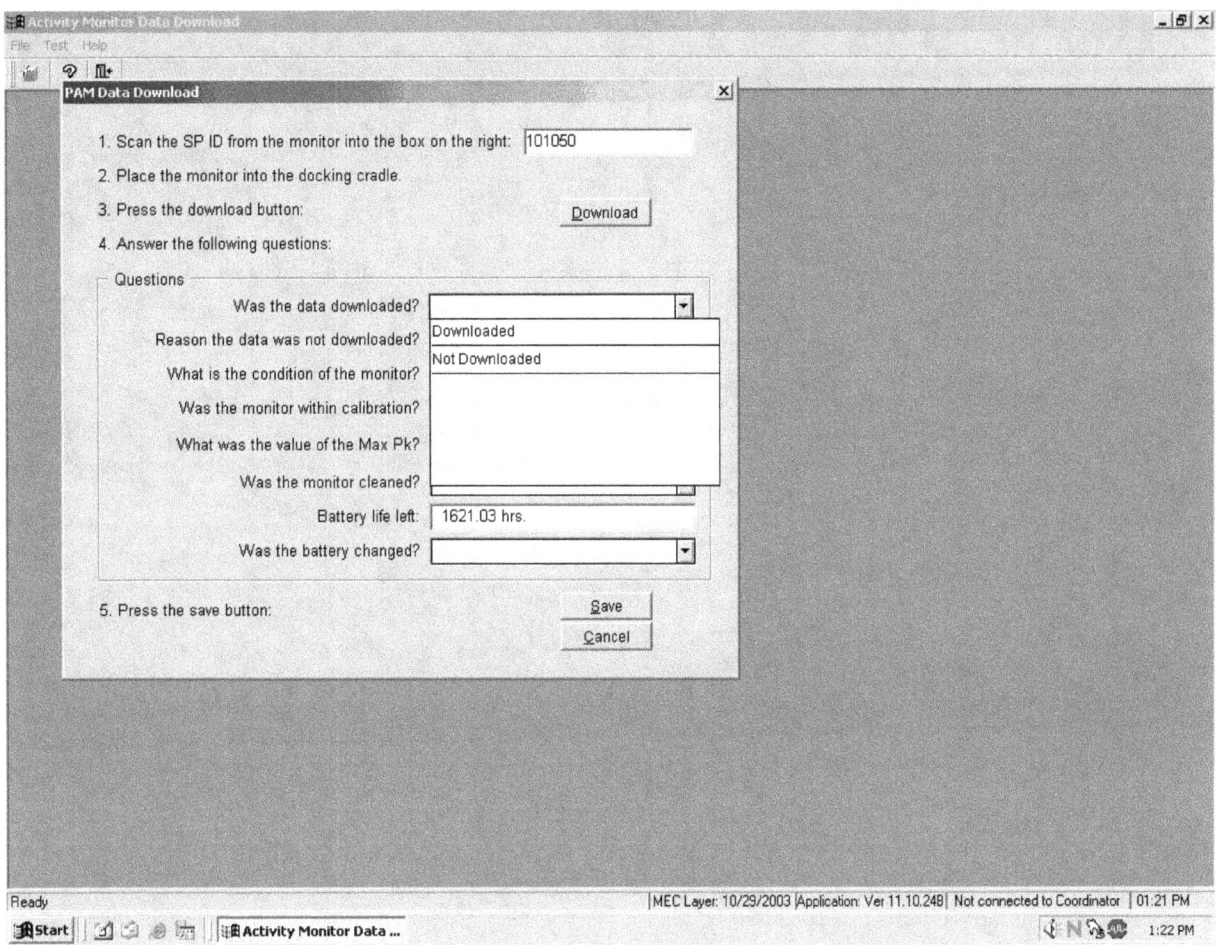

There are two possible responses to this question: Downloaded or Not Downloaded. Record the response by typing [D/d] for "Downloaded" or [N/n] for "Not Downloaded." Alternatively, use the mouse to direct the mouse arrow to the drop-down arrow on the drop-down list, left click to display the responses, and drag the mouse arrow to "Downloaded" or "Not Downloaded" and left click.

If the response to the first question is "Not Downloaded" then the second question text box is activated. Answer the second question, "Reason the data was not downloaded?"

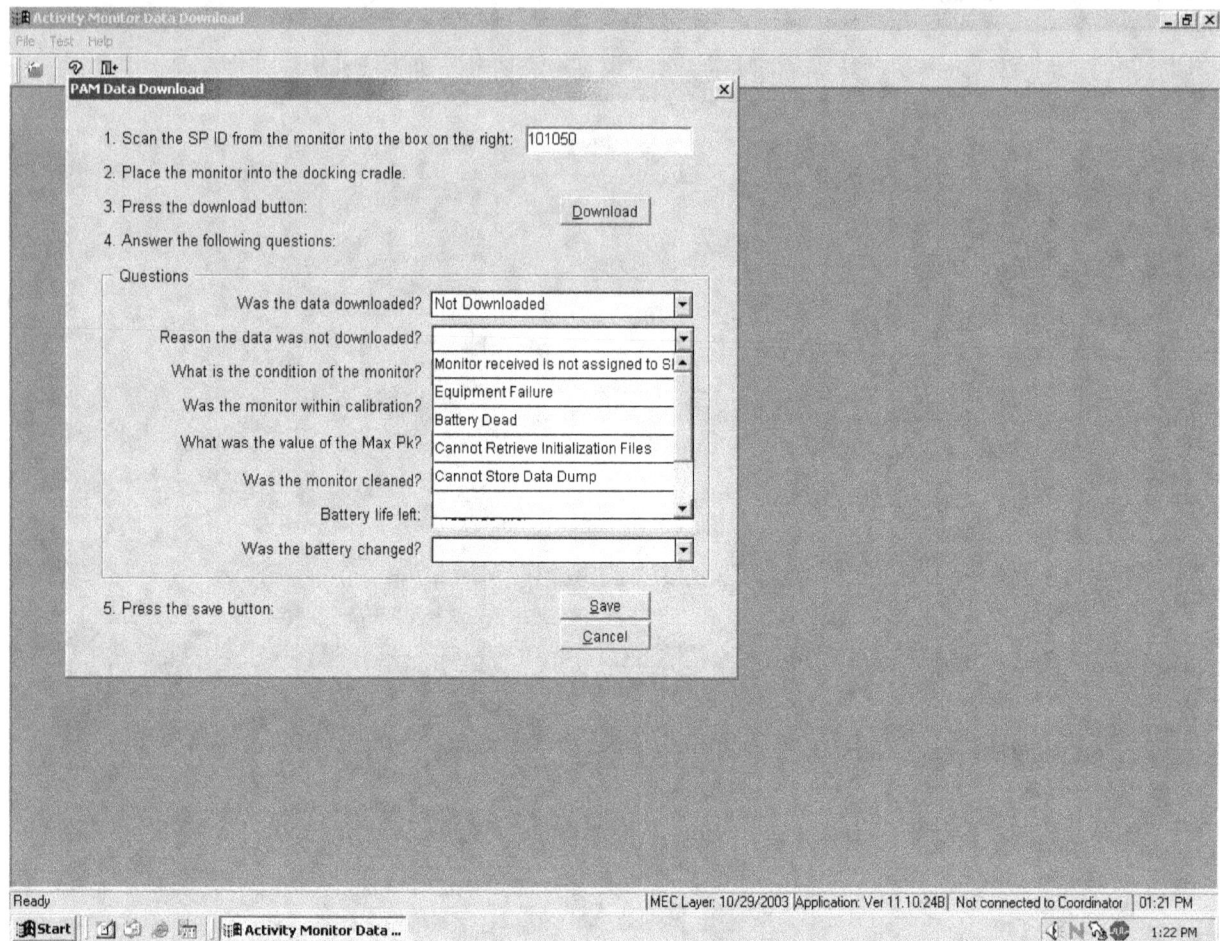

There are several reasons for a data download failure: Monitor received not assigned to SP, Equipment Failure, Battery Dead, Cannot Retrieve Initialization Files, and Cannot Store Data Dump. If the monitor fails because the RIU is broken, or the monitor is damaged beyond repair, record equipment failure. If the battery is dead, then replace the battery and repeat the data download process. If the RIU is broken, then obtain (from the warehouse), install the backup RIU, and repeat the process. If there is no backup available, then save the monitor until a replacement can be obtained. If the monitor is damaged beyond repair, then record "Equipment Failure" in the text box. Record this response by typing the first letter of the comment in the text box. Alternatively, use the mouse to direct the mouse arrow to the drop-down arrow on the drop-down list, left click to display the response, and drag the mouse arrow to the desired choice and left click.

Answer the third question, "What is the condition of the monitor?"

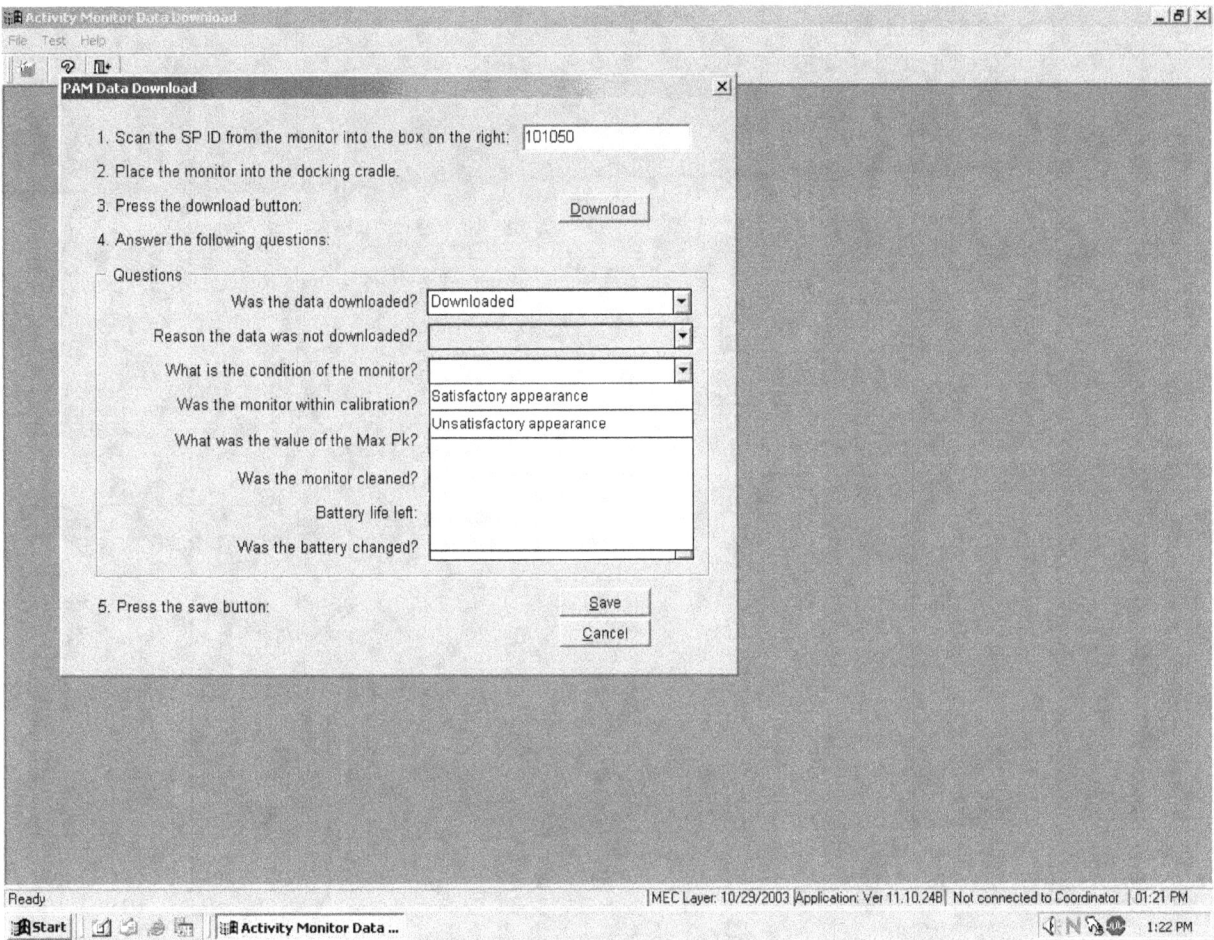

There are two possible responses to this question: Satisfactory appearance or Unsatisfactory appearance. Inspect the monitor case carefully for cracks. If the monitor case is not cracked, record "Satisfactory appearance." If the monitor case is cracked, record "Unsatisfactory appearance" and send the monitor to MTI for repair. Record the response by typing [S/s] for "Satisfactory appearance," or [U/u] for "Unsatisfactory appearance." Alternatively, use the mouse to direct the mouse arrow to the drop-down arrow on the drop-down list, left click to display the responses, and drag the mouse arrow to "Satisfactory appearance" or "Unsatisfactory appearance" and left click.

Calibrate every monitor after the data download is complete and after responding to the subsequent questions.

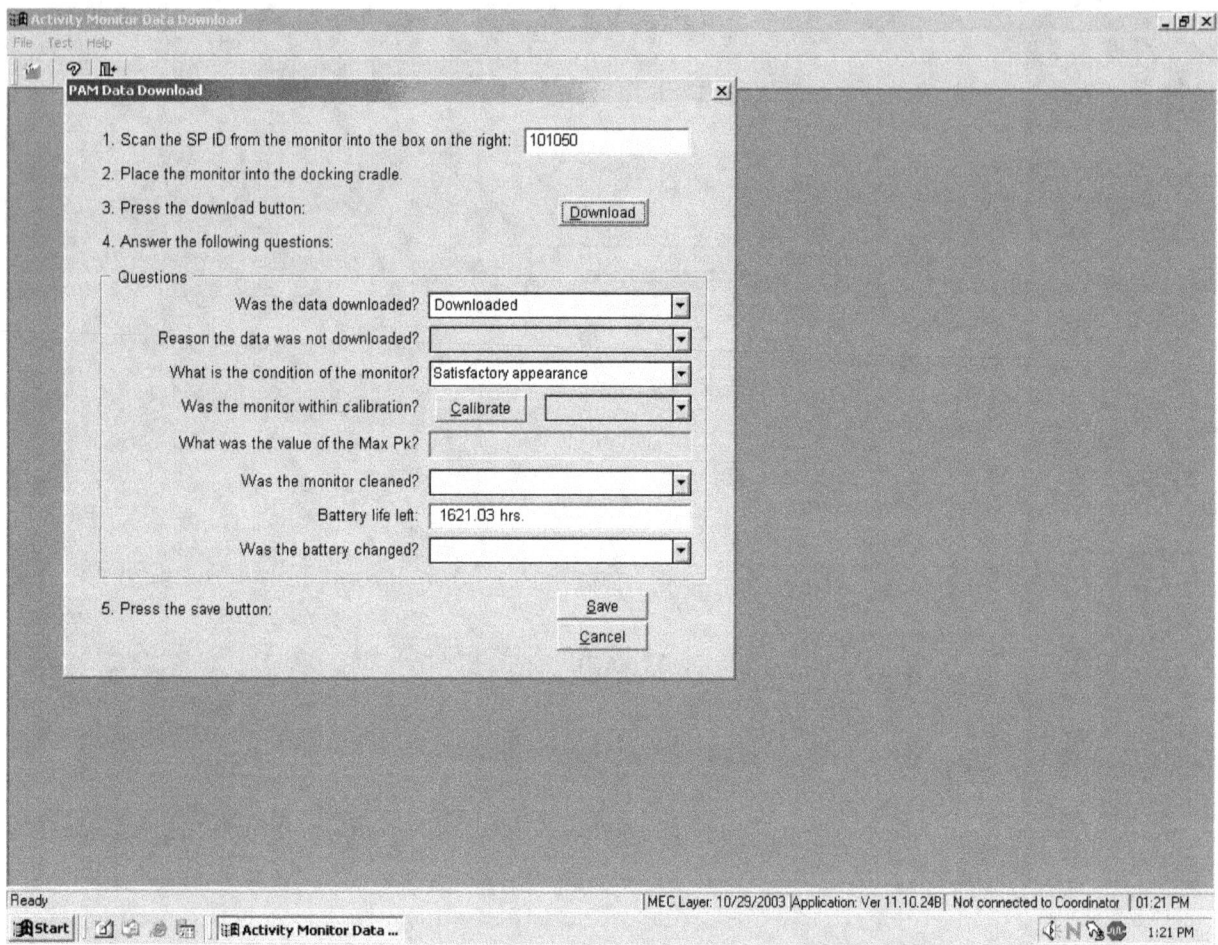

To calibrate a monitor:

1.     Position the calibration unit cradle with the open side facing the up position;

2.     Slide the monitor into the calibration cradle with the screws to the back and the smooth side toward the front and the notches down. The LED should flash red; and

3.     To begin the calibration, use the mouse to direct the mouse arrow to the Calibrate button and left click. This action launches the calibration program.

The calibration application launches when the Calibration button is selected.

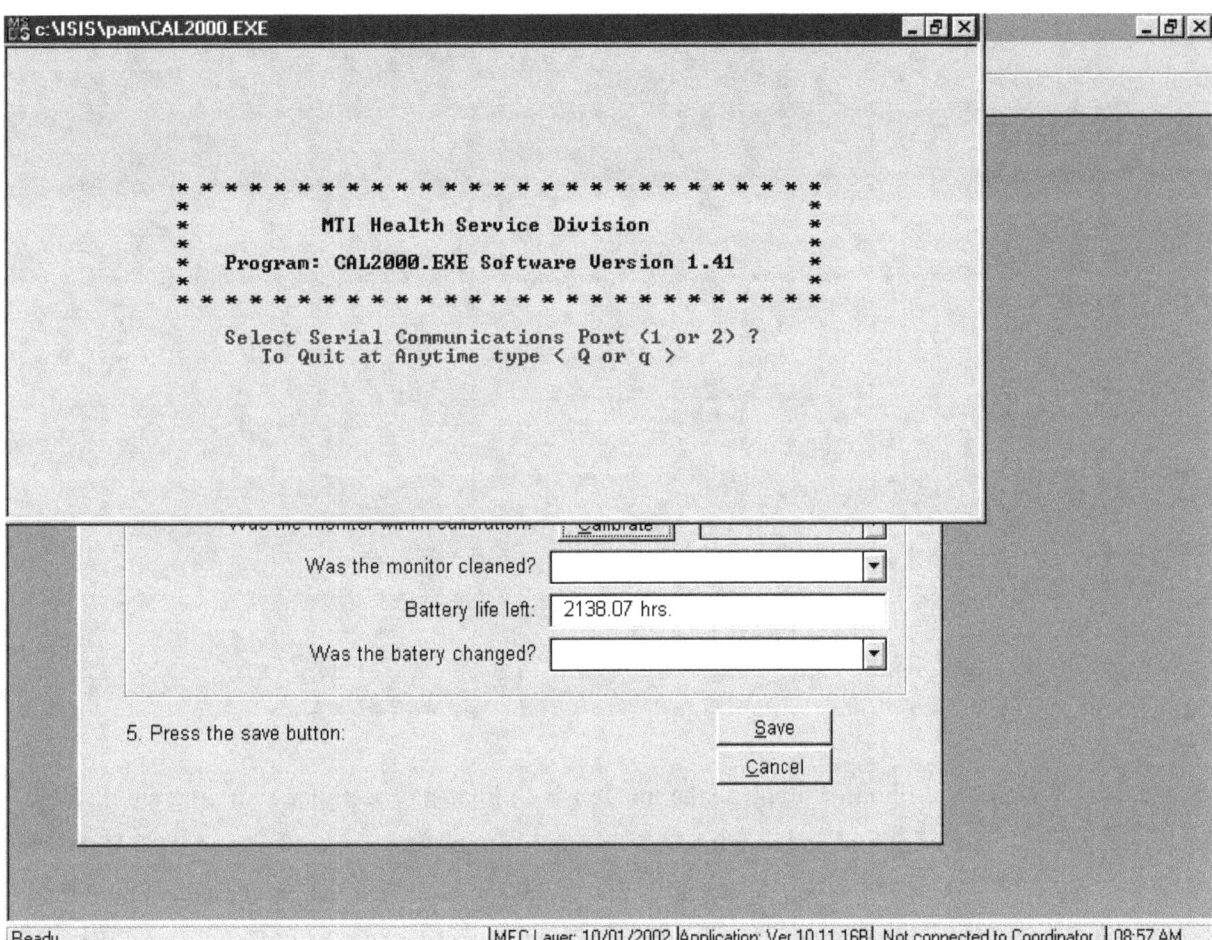

To select the Serial Communication Port number, use the keyboard to select the number "2" when the calibration program asks for the port number.

The calibration unit rotates or spins the monitor during the actual calibration.

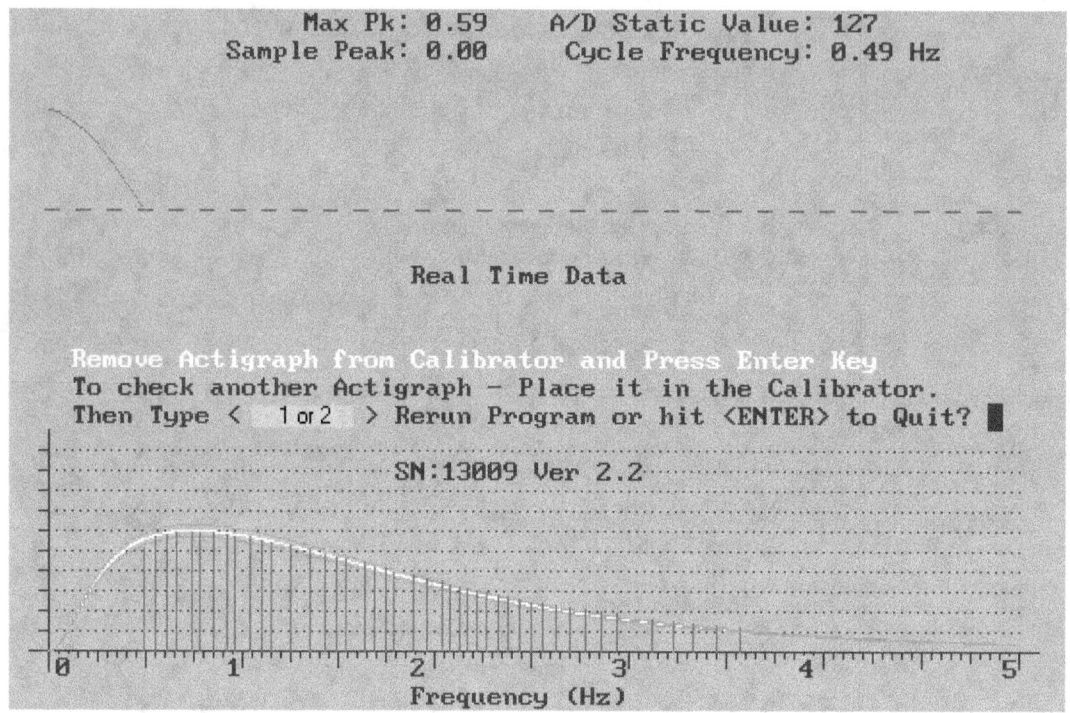

Watch the calibration graph as the monitor is calibrated. The calibration program displays a Max Pk number after the calibration is complete. This number must be between 0.57 and 0.63. If the Max Pk is between 0.57 and 0.63 then no adjustment is necessary and the monitor is calibrated. If the Max Pk is <0.57 or >0.63, then the monitor is not in calibration and must be sent to MTI for repair. Press the [Enter] key to exit the calibration program.

Answer the question, "Was the monitor within calibration?"

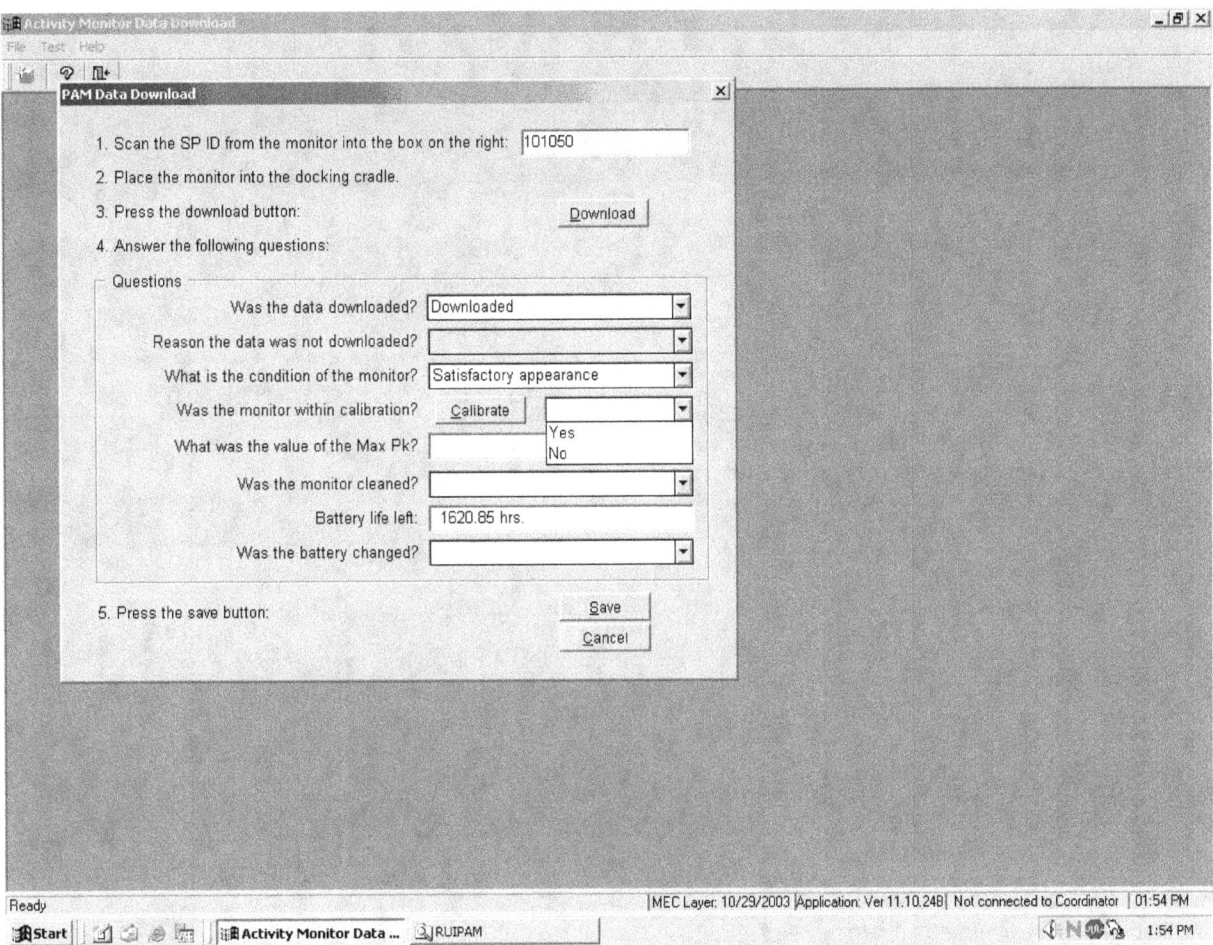

There are two possible responses to this question: Yes or No. If the Max Pk is between 0.57 and 0.63 then record "Yes." If the Max Pk is <0.57 or >0.63, then record "No." Record the responses by typing [Y/y] for "Yes," or [N/n] for "No." Alternatively, use the mouse to direct the mouse arrow to the drop-down arrow on the drop-down list, left click to display the responses, and drag the mouse arrow to "Yes" or "No" and left click.

Answer the question, "What is the value of the Max Pk?"

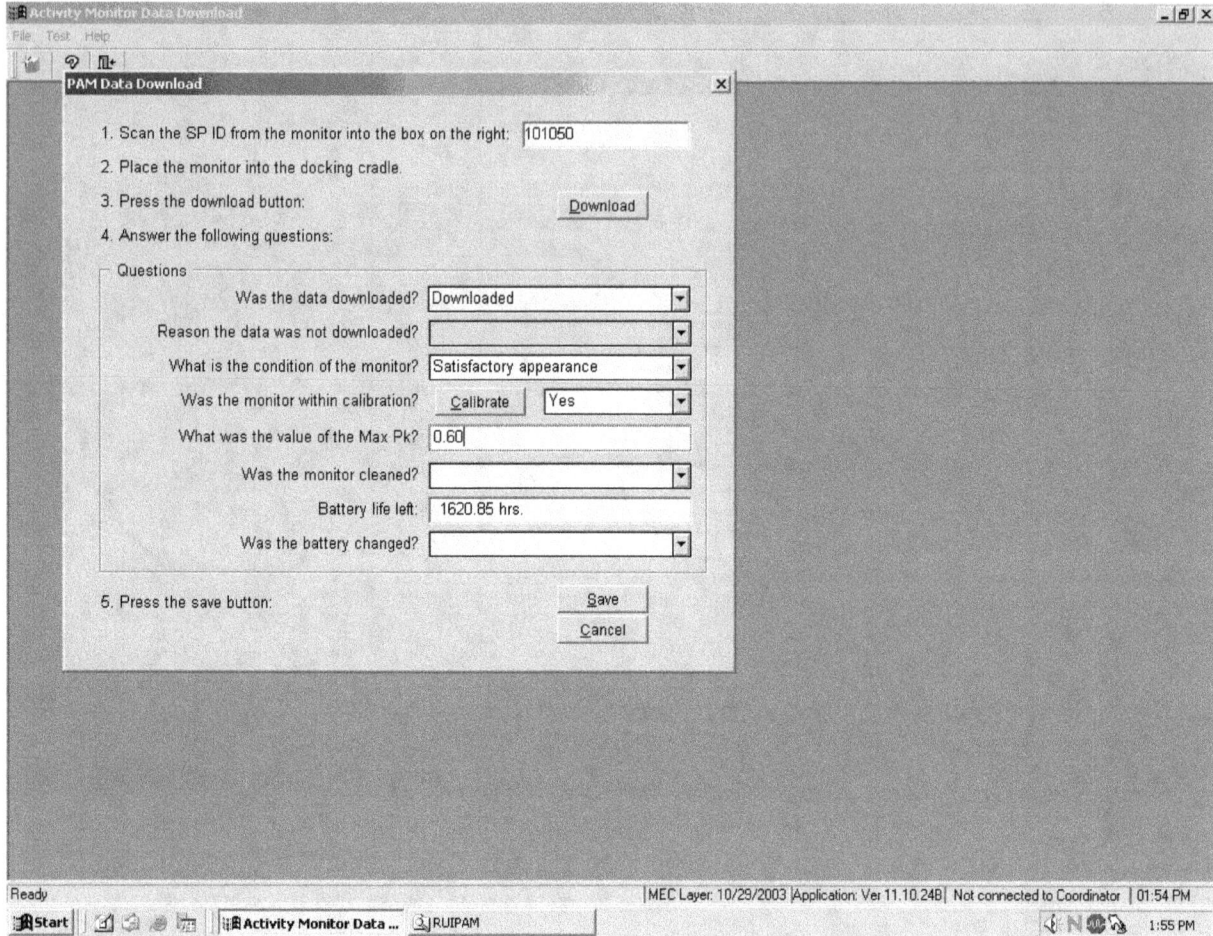

To record the value of the Max Pk in the text box, use the mouse to direct the mouse arrow to the text box and left click. Use the keyboard keys to enter a value using a X.XX format, where there is one number before the decimal and two numbers after the decimal.

Answer the question, "Was the monitor cleaned?"

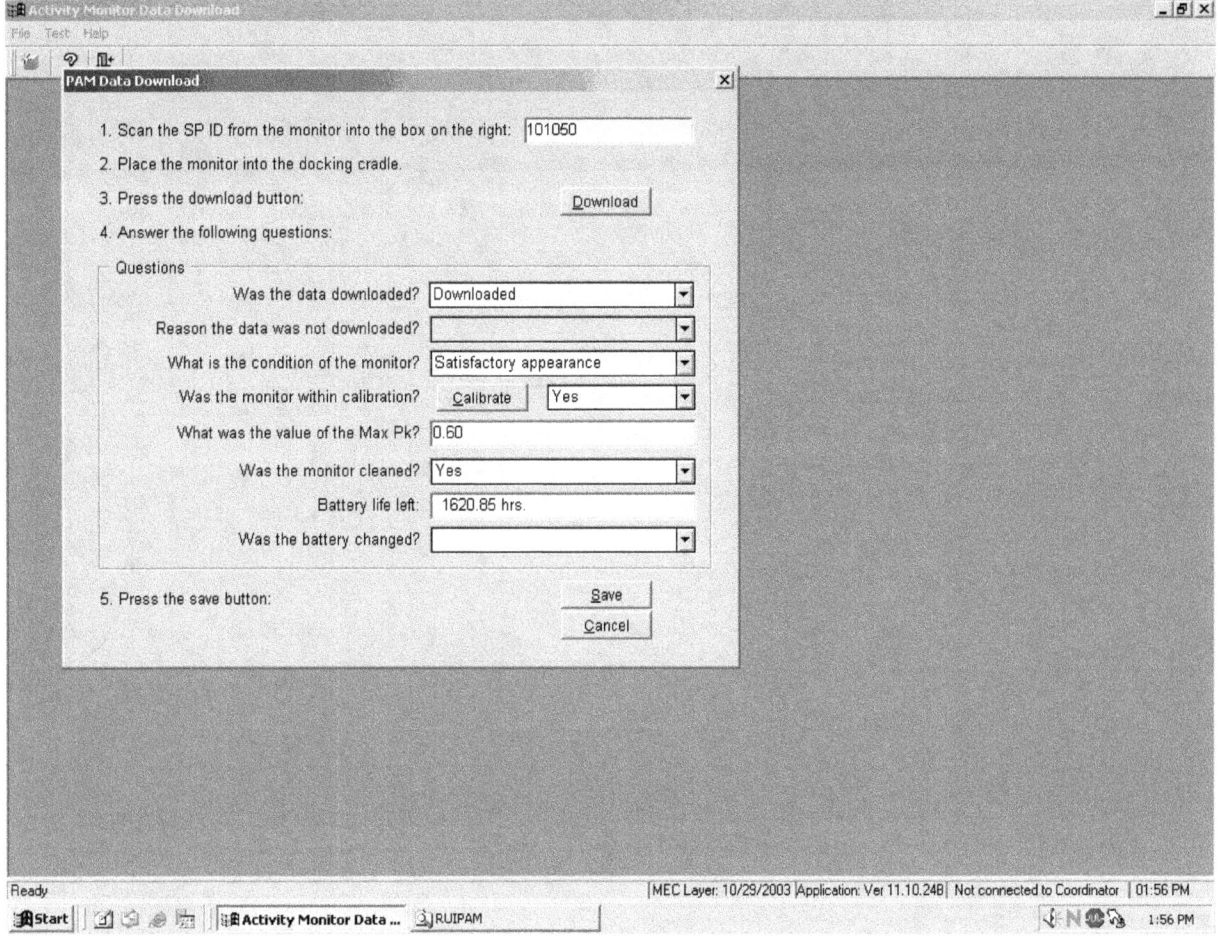

There are two possible responses to this question—Yes or No. Clean every monitor using procedures described in Section 6.14.2. Record the responses by typing [Y/y] for "Yes," or [N/n] for "No." Alternatively, use the mouse to direct the mouse arrow to the drop-down arrow on the drop-down list, left click to display the responses, and drag the mouse arrow to "Yes" or "No" and left click.

Review the number of hours displayed in the Battery life left text box.

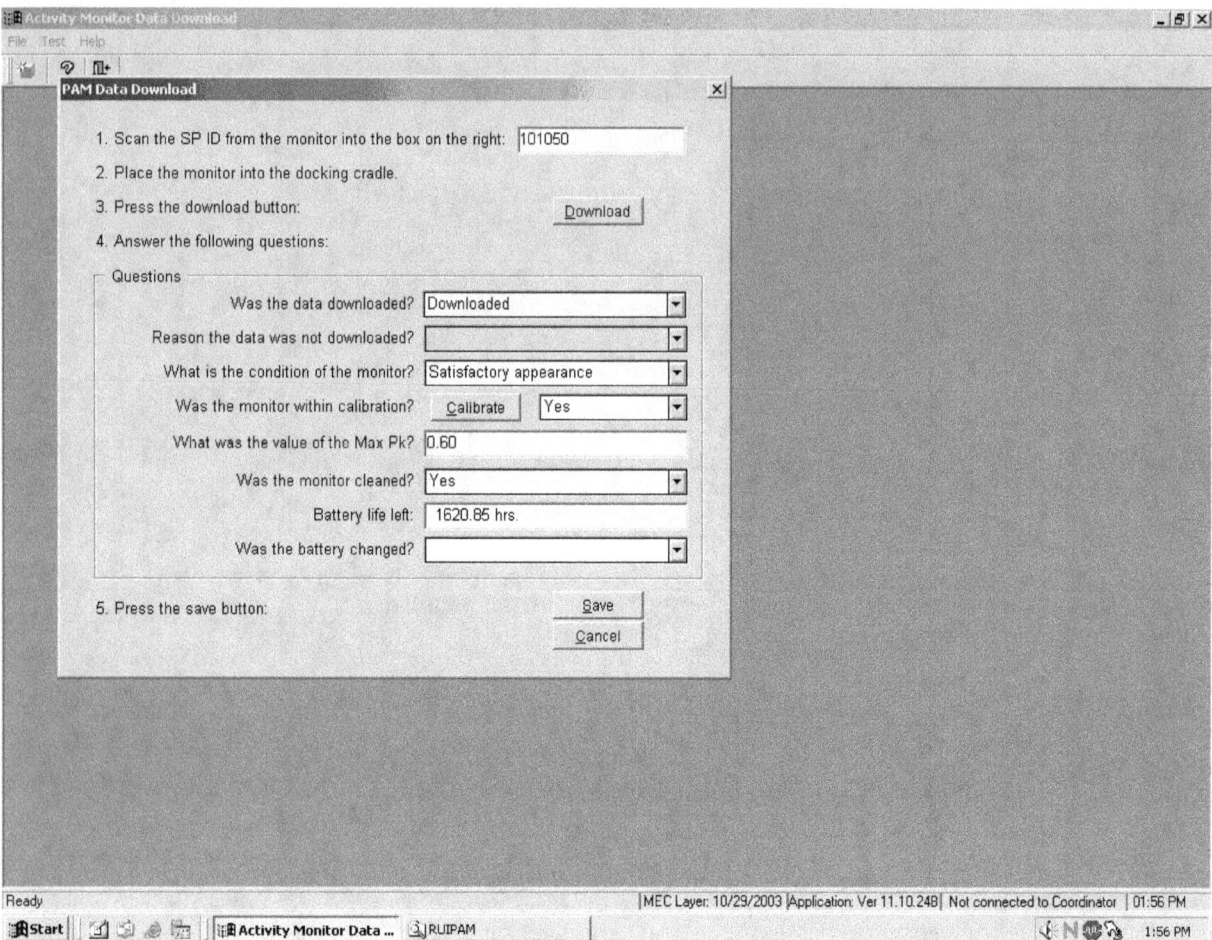

If the number of hours displayed in the Battery life left text box is less than or equal to 1,000, change the battery using procedures described in Section 6.14.1.

Answer the question, "Was the battery changed?"

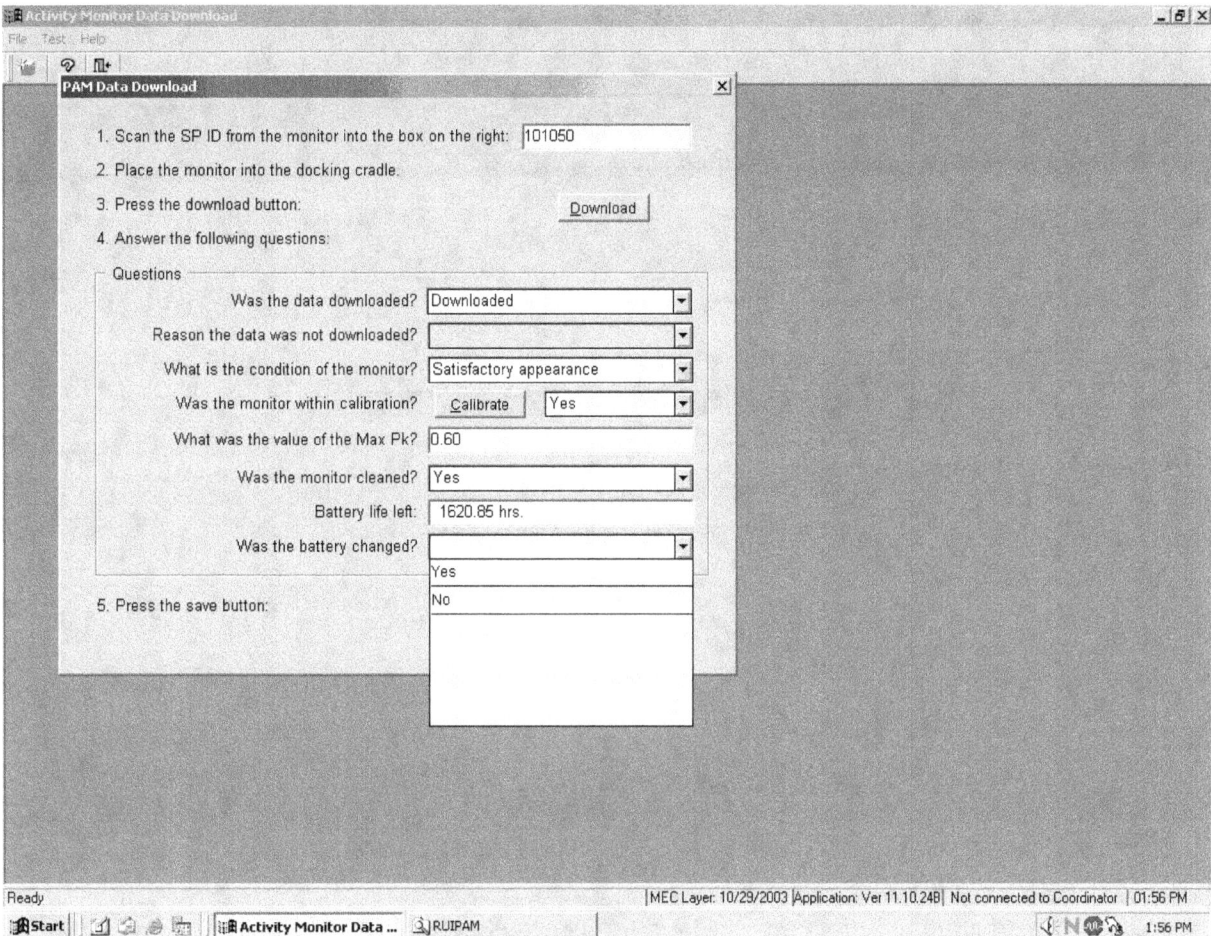

There are two possible responses to this question—Yes or No. Record the responses by typing [Y/y] for "Yes," or [N/n] for "No." Alternatively, use the mouse to direct the mouse arrow to the drop-down arrow on the drop-down list, left click to display the responses, and drag the mouse arrow to "Yes" or "No" and left click.

Save the data for this SP.

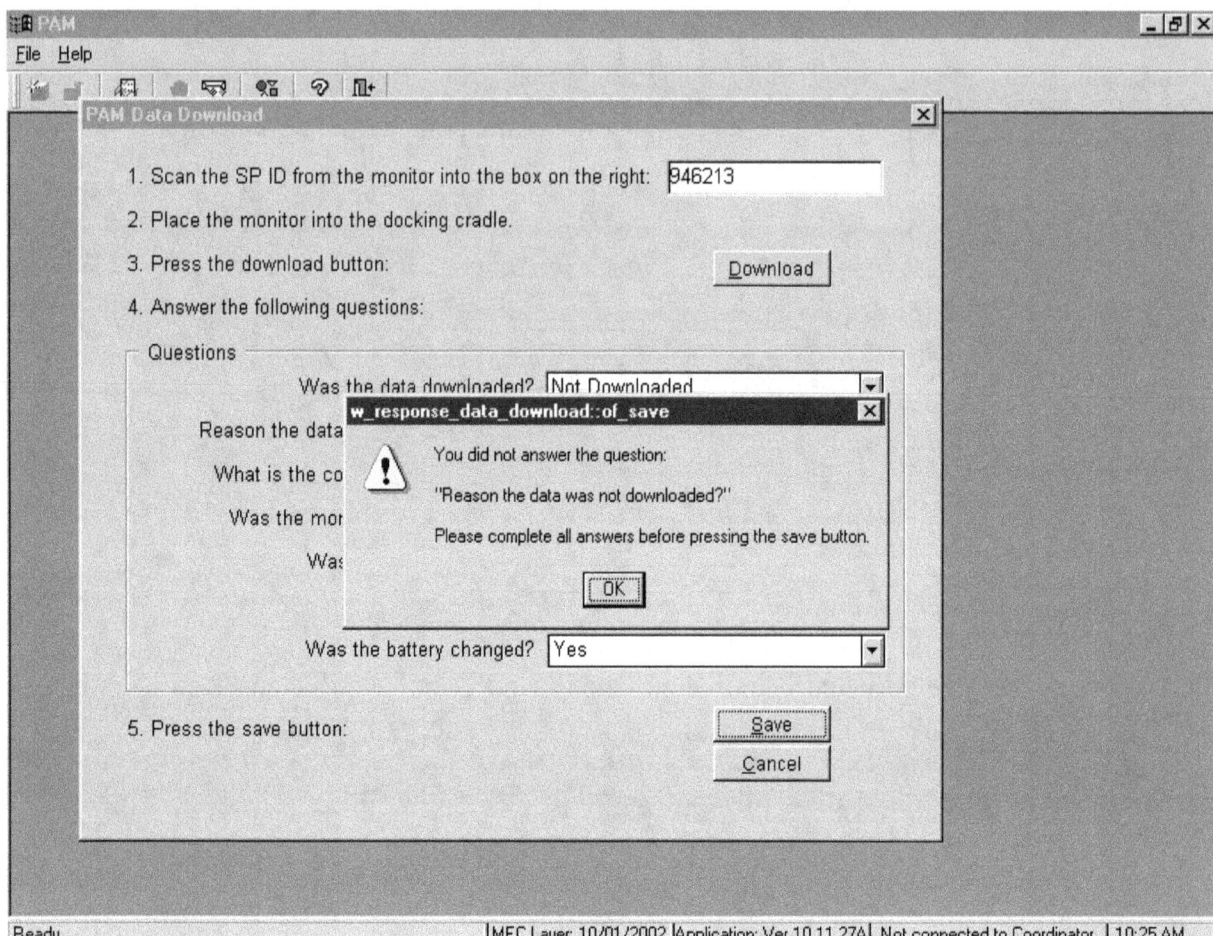

If the Save button is selected and one or more of the text boxes does not contain a response, then a warning message box displays requesting an answer to each unanswered question. To remove the warning message box, use the mouse to direct the mouse arrow to direct the mouse arrow to the OK button and left click or select [Enter].

Select the Cancel button to exit the data download and calibration process without saving any of the data to the database and to restart the process at the beginning.

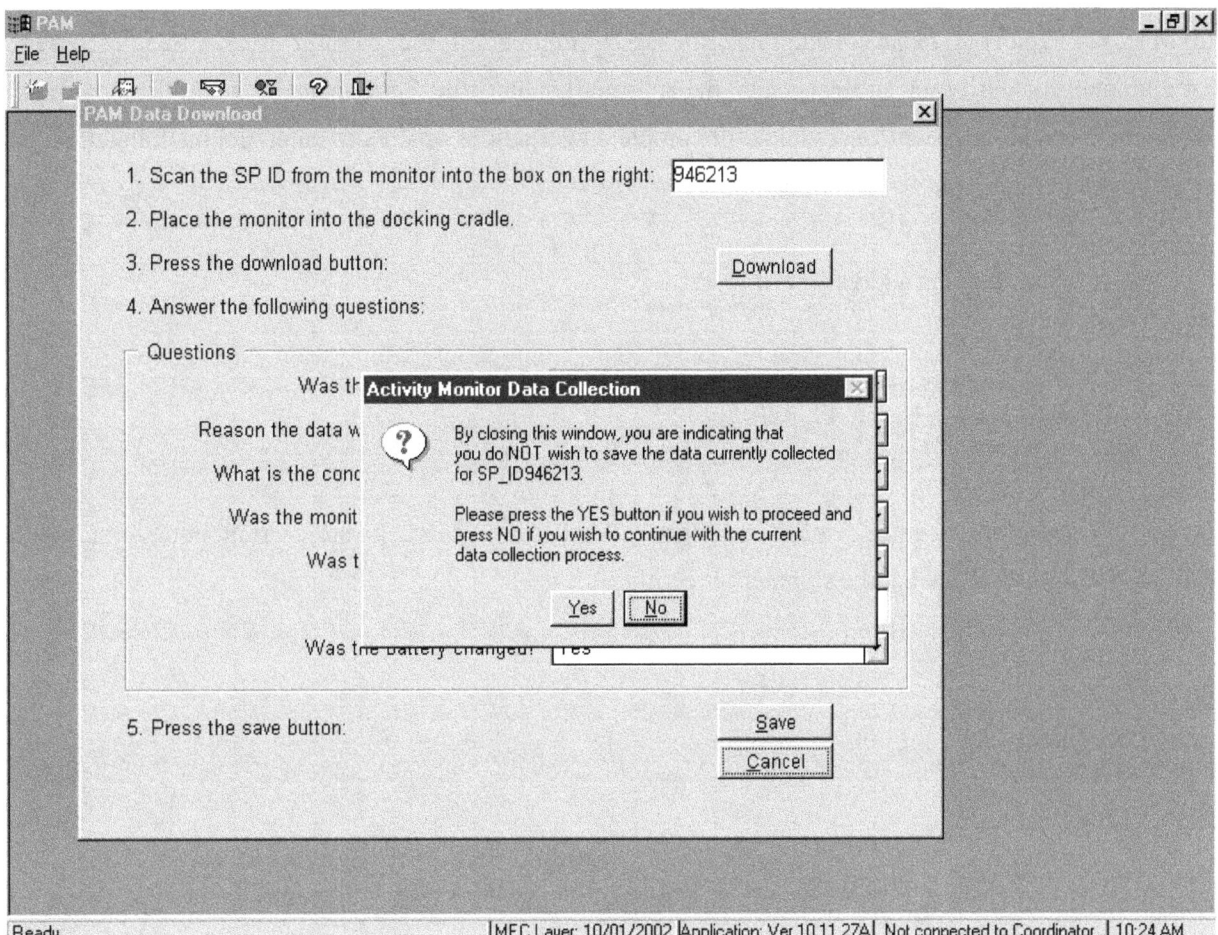

To exit the data download and calibration process without saving any of the data to the database and to restart the process at the beginning, use the mouse to direct the mouse arrow to the Yes button and left click. To continue with the data collection (data download and calibration) process, use the mouse to direct the mouse arrow to the No button and left click or select [Enter].

## 6.15     Sending Monitors for Repair or Replacement

Use the Equipment Tracking System to document the actions taken when sending a monitor to MTI for repair or replacement. Give the serial number of the monitor to the Senior Systems Programmer so that he or she can enter the information into the Equipment ID table. Reference the Equipment Tracking System User Guide for complete instructions on how to enter and track the monitors sent for repair.

The shipping address for MTI is:

Actigraph
709 Anchors Street, NW
Fort Walton Beach, FL 32548
850-244-7211

Send the monitor priority overnight to MTI using FedEx. Insure each monitor for $300.00. Call MTI to inform them that the shipment is coming.

## 6.16    English and Spanish Screenshots

English

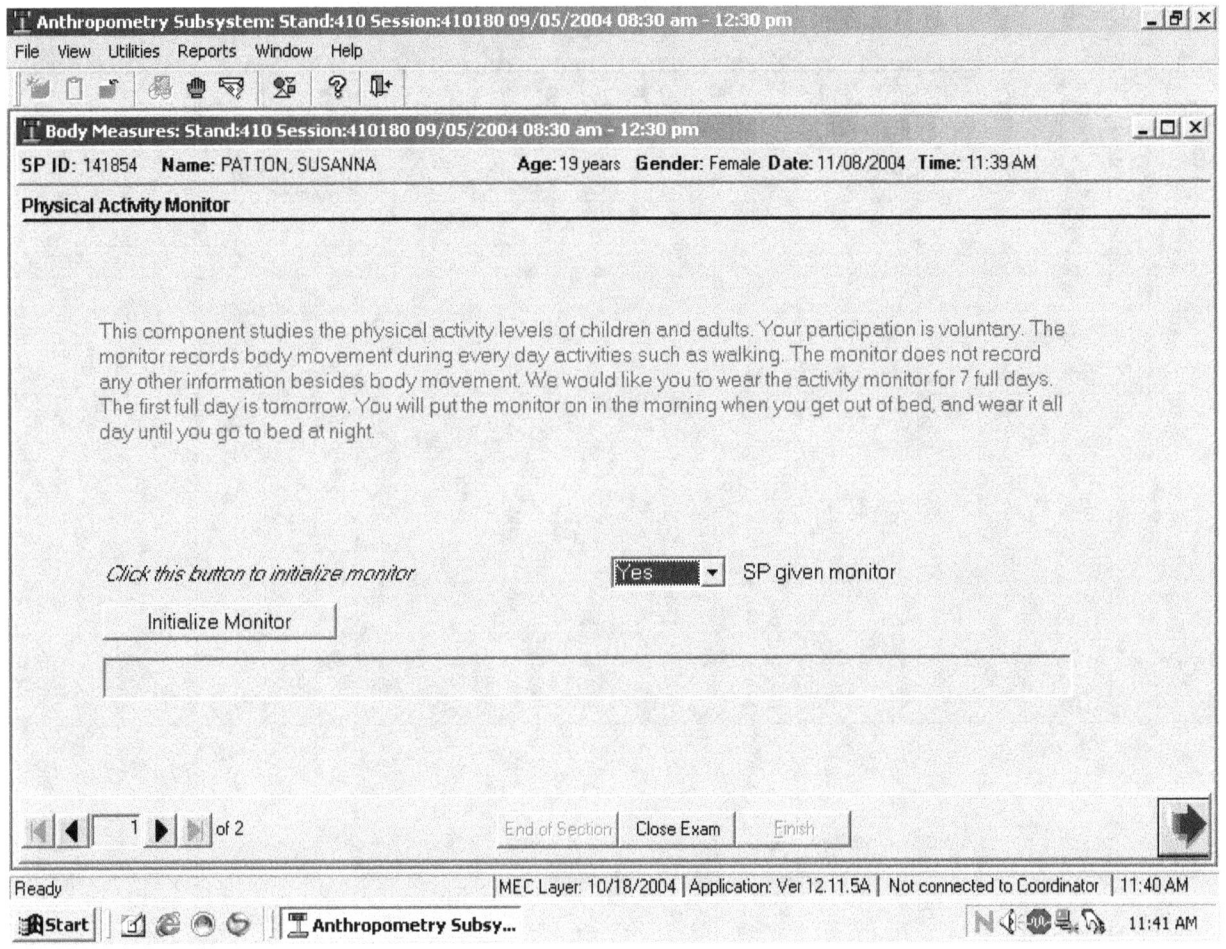

Spanish

## 6.17    References

1.  Berlin, J.A. and Colditz, G.A. (1990). A meta-analysis of physical activity in the prevention of coronary heart disease. *American Journal of Epidemiology*, 132, 612-628.

2.  Blair, S.N. and Morrow, Jr. J.R. (1998). Introduction: Cooper Institute/American College of Sports Medicine 1997 Physical Activity Intervention Conference. *American Journal of Preventative Medicine*, 15, 255-256.

3.  Janz, K.F. (1994). Validation of the CSA accelerometer for assessing children's physical activity. *Medicine and Science in Sports and Exercise*, 26, 369-75.

4.  Trost, S.G., Ward, D.S., Moorehead, S.M., Watson, P.D., Riner, W., and Burke, J. (1998). Validity of the computer science and application (CSA) activity monitor in children. *Medicine and Science in Sports and Exercise, 30, 629-33.*

5.  U.S. Department of Health and Human Services (1996). *The U.S. Surgeon General's Report on Physical Activity and Health.* SN 017-023-00196-5).

Appendix A

Body Measures Recording Form

## **Body Measures Recording Form**

**SP ID:**_____  **Stand #:**_____  **Session/Date:**_____

| MEASURES | | BIRTH + | 2MO+ | 7MO+ | 2YR+ | 4YR+ | 8YR+ |
|---|---|---|---|---|---|---|---|
| (BMXWT) | Weight | | | | | | |
| (BMXRECUM) | Recum Length | | | | | | |
| (BMXHEAD) | Head Circ | | | | | | |
| (BMXHT) | Height | | | | | | |
| (BMXHTCRA) | Ht Correction: Above Waist | | | | | | |
| (BMXHTCRB) | Ht Correction: Below Waist | | | | | | |
| (BMXLEG) | Leg Length | | | | | | |
| *Mark Midpt. of Upper Leg Length* | | | | | | | |
| (BMXCALF) | Max Calf | | | | | | |
| (BMXARML) | Upper Arm Length | | | | | | |
| *Mark Midpt. of Upper Arm Length* | | | | | | | |
| (BMXARMC) | Arm Circ | | | | | | |
| (BMXWAIST) | Waist Circ | | | | | | |
| (BMXTHICR) | Thigh Circ | | | | | | |
| (BMXTRI) | Triceps SF | | | | | | |
| (BMXSUB) | Subscap SF | | | | | | |
| | | | | | | | |
| (BMXAMP) Amputations? **Yes/No** | | | | | | | |
| If **Yes**: | | | | | | | |
| (BMXUREXT) Upper R Extremity? **Yes/No** | | | | | | | |
| (BMXUPREL) Upper R. **Above/Below** Elbow? | | | | | | | |
| (BMXULEXT) Upper L Extremity? **Yes/No** | | | | | | | |
| (BMXUPLEL) Upper L **Above/Below** Elbow? | | | | | | | |
| (BMXLOREX) Lower R Extremity? **Yes/No** | | | | | | | |
| (BMXLORKN) Lower R. **Above/Below** Knee? | | | | | | | |
| (BMXLLEXT) Lower L Extremity? **Yes/No** | | | | | | | |
| (BMXLLKNE) Lower L. **Above/Below** Knee? | | | | | | | |